The Professional Qualifying Examinations
A Survival Guide for Optometrists

D1556140

For Butterworth-Heinemann:
Publishing Director: Caroline Makepeace
Development Editor: Kim Benson
Production Manager: Yolanta Motylinska
Design: Steven Gardiner Ltd, Cambridge

The Professional Qualifying Examinations
A Survival Guide for Optometrists

Frank Eperjesi BSc (Hons) PhD MCOptom DipOrth FAAO MILTHE
Lecturer in Clinical Optometry, Division of Optometry, Aston University, Birmingham,
Research Optometrist, Neurosciences Research Institute, Aston University, Birmingham

Martin Hodgson BSc (Hons) MCOptom, Primary Care Optometrist,
North Queensland, Remote/Rural Optometrist, Townsville Aboriginal and Islander Health Service

Michelle M. Rundström BSc (Hons) MCOptom DBO
Visiting Clinical Instructor, Aston University, Optometrist and Orthoptist, London, UK

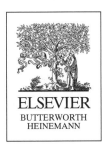

ELSEVIER
BUTTERWORTH
HEINEMANN

ELSEVIER
BUTTERWORTH
HEINEMANN

THE PROFESSIONAL QUALIFYING EXAMINATIONS   ISBN 0 7506 8845 9

Note

Medical knowledge is constantly changing. Standard safety precautions must be followed, but as new research and clinical experience broaden our knowledge, changes in treatment and drug therapy may become necessary or appropriate. Readers are advised to check the most current product information provided by the manufacturer of each drug to be administered to verify the recommended dose, the method and duration of administration, and contraindications. It is the responsibility of the practitioner, relying on experience and knowledge of the patient, to determine dosages and the best treatment for each individual patient. Neither the Publisher nor the authors/contributors assumes any liability for any injury and/or damage to persons or property arising from this publication.

First published 2004

British Library Cataloguing in Publication Data

A catalogue record for this book is available from the British Library.

Library of Congress Cataloging in Publication Data

A catalog record for this book is available from the Library of Congress.

The
publisher's
policy is to use
paper manufactured
from sustainable forests

Printed in Spain

Contents

Contributors

Simon Brooks BSc (Hons) MCOptom, Primary Care Optometrist, Barnstaple, UK

Janet Carlton BA (Open) FBDO (Hons) LVA, Dispensing Optician, Fight for Sight Optometry Clinic, City University, London, UK

Frank Eperjesi BSc (Hons) PhD MCOptom DipOrth FAAO MILTHE, Division of Optometry and Neurosciences Research Institute, Aston University, Birmingham; Examiner, College of Optometrists, UK

William Harvey MCOptom, Visiting Clinician and Director of Visual Impairment Clinic, Fight For Sight Optometry Clinic, City University, London, UK; Clinical Editor, *Optician*, UK; Professional Programme Tutor for Boots Opticians Ltd, UK; Examiner, College of Optometrists, UK

Martin Hodgson BSc (Hons) MCOptom, Optometrist, North Queensland, Australia

Ian D. Moss BSc (Hons) PhD MCOptom, Contact Lens/IT Development Director, Owl Optical Ltd, Stratford-upon-Avon, UK

John O'Donnell BSc (Hons) MCOptom FBDO, Primary Care Optometrist, London, UK

Michelle Rundström BSc (Hons) MCOptom DBO, Visiting Clinical Instructor, Aston University, Birmingham; Optometrist and Orthoptist, London, UK

Alicia Thompson FBDO SMC (Tech), ABDO Practical Examiner, SMC Examiner, Clinic Manager, Division of Optometry, Aston University, Birmingham, UK

Mary Ware BSc (Hons) MCOptom, Primary Care Optometrist, London, UK

Nu Nu Braddick BSc (Hons) MCOptom, Primary Care Optometrist, London, UK

Acknowledgements

We gratefully acknowledge those who provided contributions, help and encouragement during the writing of this book and would like to thank:

Paul Adler, Christine Astin, Danny, Gerald and Rosalee Bleetman, John Breakwell, Henry Burek, Donald Cameron, David Cartwright, Jason Clarke, Sangeeta Desai, Andy Diddams, Keith Edwards, Robert Fletcher, Charles Greenwood, Neelam and Anil Gupta, Ashley Hannigan, Gill Hardy, Berry Harley, Mark Harmer, Tazeen Iqbal, Brian Keefe, Zara Komall, Jerry Lewis, Robert Linsky, Ian Maclean, Aileen McClean, Judith Morris, D Morris, Satpal Multani, Urszula Mosdorf-Skrzeczkowska, Henry Obstfeld, Greg Parker, Linda Penny, Joan Pugh, Zerin and Alin Razzaque, Stuart Rose, B Rughani, Nick Rumney, Lynne Speedwell, Paul Stratton, Ian Truelove, Phil Turner, Fred Giltrow-Tyler, and J Zajaczkowska.

Special thanks to Richard Allen and Ushma Desai for comments on an earlier version of this book.

Introduction

This book is a guide for undergraduate students applying for a pre-registration position and for pre-registration optometrists taking the College of Optometrists (CO) Part II Professional Qualifying Examinations (PQEs). The book should be used in conjunction with all communications and publications available from the CO relating to the pre-registration year and the PQEs.

If you are wondering what happened to Part I, you may be glad to read that your Optometry degree is Part I as long as you obtained at least a lower second-class degree in Optometry from a university based in the United Kingdom. If you obtained a third class or pass degree in Optometry then you will have to sit Part I PQEs and pass before being allowed to take Part II PQEs. We have very little experience of Part I PQEs and therefore they are not covered in this book. However, one thing we do know is that Part I PQEs are extremely difficult and rarely passed, probably because they are taken by people who did not make the most of their learning opportunities while at university and therefore do not have the requisite knowledge of basic optometric theory and lack clinical skills. Needless to say, it is better to graduate with at least a lower second-class Optometry degree and avoid Part I PQEs. If you have an Optometry degree from another country then contact the CO for information on PQE requirements.

The pre-registration year is hard work for little financial reward and the examinations at the end of it are difficult. We urge you to make the most of the pre-registration year and accumulate as much experience as possible. Use every resource at your disposal. This will give you more confidence in the examinations and benefit you in your future career. The rewards for successful candidates are well worth all the work.

The PQEs are a difficult and daunting set of examinations. You should not assume that because you have managed to pass a degree in Optometry that you will automatically become a competent practitioner. The PQEs assess your competence in clinical practice and in combining practical skills with a sound knowledge of theory. To paraphrase a North American guide for examiners in optometry: 'The examiner represents an interface between an individual's desire (often perceived as a right) to practise his or her chosen profession, and the need of the public to be protected'.

The CO states that its formal objective is: 'The maintenance for the public benefit of the highest possible standards of professional competence and conduct.' Therefore, the standards required by examiners are (rightly) very high. The examiners and the PQEs are often criticized by candidates. Some critical comments seem justified, though candidates who complain or appeal against certain decisions usually find this course of action unproductive. The purpose of this guide is not to criticize or defend the PQEs; our aims are to help the undergraduate find a pre-registration placement and then to pass the PQEs.

Shortly after this book was written we discovered that the CO had plans to change the PQEs. At the time of publication these plans were still under discussion, but it seems likely that the current examination format will change in spring 2006. Trainees entering the pre-registration year in Autumn 2005 will undergo more in-practice assessment, a process that will involve their supervisor and a CO-appointed assessor. Once the in-practice assessment has been completed satisfactorily, a series of practical assessments will take place over one day at an assessment centre. The exact nature of these practical assessments and the topics covered has yet to be decided.

We stress that it is important to note for yourself any changes to the examination format that have been made since the publication of this guide. Also we cannot guarantee that you will pass your PQEs after reading this book and following our advice, but we are sure that you will stand a better chance. It is best to assume that the past examination questions listed at the end of each chapter in Part 2 of this book will probably not be asked in your examinations.

The publishers would be very grateful to receive any comments on this first edition of guide and any advice or material for future editions.

We hope that you find this book useful. Good luck.

FE, MH *and* MMR

How to use this book

It should be obvious which parts of the book should be referred to at any particular time. However, we have included this short section in the hope that it will help save your valuable time. The book is presented in a logical order, from applying for a pre-registration position to finally sitting the examinations.

If you have bought this book and already have a pre-registration place then Part 1 can be ignored and you can go straight to Part 2 now. However, if you are yet to secure a pre-registration position then read both parts and carry on below.

At the beginning of the second year at your university it will be useful to read Chapter 1, which aims to help you to choose the right environment for your pre-registration year. Perhaps also glance at Chapter 2, which will give you an idea of what paperwork you will receive from the CO during your final university year in preparation for the start of your pre-registration year. After securing a pre-registration position, we advise you to forget the PQEs until you graduate from university. Concentrate on your final year examinations!

Just before you start your pre-registration year read Chapters 2 to 5, which explain what to expect in the year ahead and give advice on how to make the best of your time. Hopefully you won't need to refer to Chapter 6, but most candidates do have at least one examination to re-sit. This chapter offers advice if you are unsuccessful in one or more examinations after the first sitting.

Work through Chapters 7 to 16 on the individual examination subjects. These chapters advise on preparation for individual examinations including recommendations about activities, e.g. hospital visits and factory tours, which we strongly advise you to arrange during the year. These chapters are all of a similar format. They have the following sub-headings:

1 What does the CO say? This is taken from the CO syllabus, sometimes with our comments added in italics.
2 The examination format – our description of what may happen to you in the examinations.

3 What do the examiners say? Responses to questionnaires sent to examiners asking questions about the PQEs. We have included the best comments for each section.
4 Help and advice – this is about preparing for the subject during the pre-registration year and taking the examinations.
5 Past exam questions – taken from candidates following their exams and also from examiners. These will be useful for indicating the types of question you *might* be asked.
6 Suggested reading – but also refer to the CO list sent to you early in the pre-registration year.

The chapters in this book have been compiled by different authors so formats may vary slightly and there may be some repetition; this will serve to highlight important points.

Each chapter in Part 2 is a practical guide to preparing for and sitting each PQE, and so contains little information about the theory and practice of the subject. You will learn all that during university and the pre-registration year: we did not want to make this book into a monster text!

PART 1

A guide to the pre-registration year

1

Applying for a pre-registration position

At some point during your second or final year at university you will be applying for a position as a pre-registration optometrist. Many students apply at the beginning of the final academic year in the hope that they will be able to pick and choose the job that will suit them, although we have noticed that more and more students are applying for positions during their second year at university. Some students prefer to apply at the end of the final year after completing their university exams. This approach allows you to concentrate on finals, but often means that there may be little or no choice in the type and location of a pre-registration position and we do not advocate leaving your pre-registration applications until this time.

The pre-registration year can either be spent in the hospital eye service (HES), in an independent private practice, or working for a multiple company; there are also a few places in university optometry departments. Each type of position has advantages and disadvantages when compared to the others. Later in this chapter we will compare the options in more detail. It is absolutely vital that during the pre-registration year you gain experience in all areas of optometric practice, so it is important that you spend some time away from your chosen option and work in other environments. It is also important that you have time to attend ophthalmology, orthoptic and low vision clinics, industrial sites, spectacle and contact lens manufacturers, and indeed any other place with relevance to optometric practice.

It is worth remembering when applying for a pre-registration position that it will be your vehicle to preparing for the PQEs. Much of this preparation needs to be completed in the short period from August to March, so your prospective employer will need to be well prepared to meet your requirements for equipment, guidance and time off for visits and revision. Later in this chapter we will give advice on dealing with the interview. This gives you an opportunity to ask the interviewer questions to make certain that the pre-registration experience you need can be provided.

First you need to choose which type of pre-registration position you would like and its locality. At some stage in the second or final year of your university course, representatives from some of the multiples may give presentations at your university describing the pre-registration year they offer. Most students will have visited a hospital optometry department during the course of their studies and some students will have some experience of optometric practice from weekend or vacation work. It is always worthwhile contacting your university careers office for support with the application process. Careers officers are used to advising optometry students and can help with CV and cover letter preparation as well as with developing interview techniques. We have included some basic hints and tips on writing cover letters and CVs below.

WRITING A COVER LETTER

Job-hunting is an uncertain activity at the best of times, and when faced with a high volume of applications, a recruiter will look for any reason to reduce the pile – which is why you need a cover letter that works hard for you.

Properly constructed, it can be an attention-grabbing document that introduces you to a prospective employer as interesting, enthusiastic, suitable for the job, and spurs them to look at your CV. They can, however, be challenging to write and it's easy to go off-beam. The guidelines outlined below will help make your cover letters more targeted and effective.

Structure and content

Cover letters should be concise and consist of no more than four paragraphs. They should comprise:

First paragraph: Specify the job you are applying for and where you heard of it. If it was a referral, mention the person's name.

Middle paragraph(s): This forms the centre of your pitch to the recruiter and needs to summarize the key aspects of your CV in an original and clever way.

Open with a positive statement – you want them to stay awake, don't you? Explain how your skills, education and experience qualify you for the advertised role.

Demonstrate that you have thoroughly researched the company and understand its dealings. The trade and business press is a handy way of finding out more about the trends and issues in a particular sector. In the unlikely event that you are unable to track down relevant information, request background information from the company – it will make you seem genuine and add to your credibility.

Bullet-point them if there are three or more points. Resist the temptation to exaggerate, as you are likely come unstuck at interview. Steer clear of adjectives and unsupported value judgements, such as: 'I am an energetic and motivated team player'. They don't mean anything and won't help your case.

Final paragraph: Reaffirm your interest and suitability for the position in a few well-chosen words. Conclude the letter politely and indicate how you intend to follow up.

Presentation and style

Unless a handwritten letter is requested, use a word processor and a clear, legible font such as Times New Roman – it looks more professional. Keep your letter to one side of A4 and ensure the paper stock is white and of high quality – some organizations are scanning cover letters and CVs into their databases so clean typefaces and sharp printing are essential to minimize the risk of it being misread. Make sure the layout is clear and uncluttered so easily legible. Make it easy for the reader to get in touch by prominently featuring your contact details. Include telephone, mobile and e-mail details in addition to your address. This will also provide a useful back-up should your letter and CV become separated. If it is a speculative letter, customize it so the reader knows you are not sending their company the same one you have sent to ten other employers.

The tone should be formal, but be yourself – you want to sound natural, not as though you've copied a template from a careers website. Write concisely and restrict the number of sentences in each paragraph to four or five, varying the length of sentences to alter the tempo but generally keeping them short.

Finally, don't blow it

Applications are frequently rejected for spelling and grammatical errors. So never rely on your own proofreading capabilities – ask a friend or colleague to cast an eye over your letter. They can also act as a sounding board.

A convincing cover letter is the one that demonstrates the candidate has a genuine interest in the company and has done some additional research. Obtaining current information about the target company, for example, will give you a greater understanding, and enable you to explain how your skills and experience can fully support the organization's goals, or how you are compatible with the company's values.

Career sites that offer standard templates for writing cover letters can be useful in focusing you on the sort of information that you need to provide to a prospective employer. However, cover letters should always be tailored to a particular job, so, sending a generic covering letter will not enable you to demonstrate that you can actually meet the requirements of a specific role and/or company.

Cover letter top tips

- Present key aspects of your CV succinctly
- Keep to one side of A4
- Limit the number of paragraphs to no more than four
- Support accomplishments with figures
- Avoid adjectives and adverbs that are not quantifiable.

WRITING A CV

Tailor your CV to the job Employers are on the look-out for candidates who best fit their organization and position. Your CV needs to key into the organization and the position for which you are applying with greater accuracy. The CV you submit to an independent practice should be different from that submitted to a multiple.

Never let your CV go over two pages According to one source, 60 per cent of the first page of a CV registers on a first read and only 40 per cent of the second page. Such a diminishing return is bad news, but demonstrates that page three really will not be worth writing. It is also unlikely that your prospective employer will want to employ someone who cannot be concise.

Keep it relevant The CV is intended to get you to the next stage of application – the interview. It is not intended to give a full picture of you as a person. At this stage the employer wants to identify individuals with the skills and aptitude for the job. Present the picture of a competent and professional applicant and don't go overboard with unnecessary details.

Pay attention to structure CVs contain a combination of the following elements:

- Contact details
- Employment history
- Training and development undertaken
- Education and qualifications
- Personal details
- Referees

In the vast majority of cases, following this order will enable you to tell a good story about yourself through your CV. Be sure to summarize parts of your CV in order to emphasize your most current and relevant experience.

Don't bury your talent Make sure your best qualities and achievements are there on page one, ready to grab attention. Don't meander through your career expecting the reader to wait until the end for a reason to interview you. Let this dictate the structure of your CV, determining whether your employment history should come before your education and qualifications.

Concentrate on your achievements Focus on projects you initiated and those to which you made a significant contribution. Be clear and concise about the outcomes of your work. Stating your responsibilities does not show you are a good worker, simply that you had those responsibilities. Where possible, illustrate how your work has resulted in achievements beyond identified targets. Show how you have brought value to the organization that cannot be described through facts and figures, i.e. increased employee satisfaction, increased teamwork, decreasing hierarchical structures.

The obvious stuff (and so easy to overlook!)

Be honest and factual Don't elaborate on your achievements or try to tell your reader what to think through use of adjectives. Your reader is less likely to think your record is 'impressive' if you say it is.

Check and double check spelling and grammar Use a dictionary if you have any doubts. Spell checkers are not foolproof and will change your name if you're not paying attention. Get your CV read by someone else before you send it off – they don't need to know anything about the job you're applying for, just provide feedback on how you come across.

Throughout your CV try to avoid the following:

Repeated use of 'I' Or any other phrase, particularly when describing your achievements.

Jargon Optometric jargon may be necessary to show you know your area, but don't overdo it. For some appointments, your CV will be read by human resources personnel or administrative support staff who may not be familiar with this vocabulary. Explain your worth in everyday terms.

Humour A quick gag wastes space and gives the impression you aren't taking the application or yourself seriously. Wait until the interview to allow your personality to show. It is also far easier to judge another person's sense of humour in a face-to-face situation.

Gaps While employers may not expect a continuous career progression through the school or college and university, they will question time periods which are left unaccounted for. Don't be afraid to explain career breaks – better to do this than raise your reader's suspicions.

Too much detail You don't need to list every single day's training you have received or absolutely everything you did in a certain job. Keep it relevant, keep it focused. Similarly, don't go overboard with personal interests. Too much extra-curricula activities may worry an employer as to how much work you're planning to do for them. The more information you give on your CV, the more material your prospective employer has to use against you at the interview stage. Make sure they can only ask you what you want to be asked.

CV top tips

- Less is more – be concise and interest your reader
- Tailor your CV – according to the position you are after
- Don't use humour – save the quips for later
- Get a second (third and even fourth) opinion
- Presentation is the key. Use good quality paper, a single clear font (no smaller than size 12), good-sized margins and well laid out. Make sure these elements are also present in your cover letter. If you're sending your CV in electronic form, use a text file (.txt), Word 95 file or earlier. Newer files may not be readable by employers' systems
- Be comfortable with your CV. Is it who you are
- Don't send a photo unless requested
- Make sure it is clear how to contact you. If you don't want them calling you at work, give them an effective alternative.

Note This cover letter and CV advice was written by Simon Kent and originally published in *Personnel Today*. We thank the editor for allowing us to reproduce this material here.

COMPLETING APPLICATION FORMS

All the multiples and most of the hospitals will ask you to fill out an application form. These will vary in format from one company to the next but often they cover similar ground. We have provided some bad and good examples of how to answer those awkward questions dealing with topics like demonstrating leadership and teamwork.

1 Describe a situation where you demonstrated leadership

Bad example I was elected to the position of president of the Optics Society during my second year at university. The society consisted of 30 members with a five-person committee. We set objectives for the year that had to be achieved by the committee. I had to effectively manage the committee, which was a hard task but necessary for success.

Good example I was elected to the position of president of the Optics Society during my second year at university. The society consisted of 30 members with a five-person committee. My objectives were to double the number of members; increase the number of social events, and increase awareness of the eye care amongst the university students. In order to meet these targets I had to motivate the committee, and held regular team meetings to check we were achieving our objectives. By the end of the year our objectives were fulfilled and I was particularly thrilled that the membership had risen to 120.

2 Give an example of a team you have been in. What was your role in the team? How did the team work together? What was the outcome?

Bad example Last year I was involved in an expedition as part of the Duke of Edinburgh award scheme. Five of us met to plan our route over Exmoor and to allot roles. The weather was bad and one of the party injured his foot, but after much effort we completed the expedition successfully.

Good example Last year, when working for the Duke of Edinburgh gold award, five of us undertook an expedition on Exmoor in December. We each had specific roles that we decided to take, mine being to organize food supplies. Though we were keen to carry as little weight as possible, I pointed out the need not simply to provide food for the expected duration of the trip, but to carry some emergency rations in case of delay. In the event one of the team had a bad fall and we had to take turns to help support him, while battling against wind and rain. We were extremely grateful for our extra food during the inevitable delay in reaching our destination.

Application top tips

- Do your homework
- Tailor your application
- Provide detailed evidence
- Make sure it looks professional and reads well
- Create a positive impression
- Structure your responses to questions very carefully
- Always ask someone else to read your application form before sending it
- Do remember to visit your careers office while at university to get expert help with cover letter and CV writing. Your future could depend on it.

The following Sections 1.1 to 1.3 describe in more detail the three main options for a pre-registration year position. We have included comments from supervisors and recruitment personnel in each. The comments are taken from questionnaires that asked about the requirements of their particular organization and the advantages offered to successful applicants.

1.1 HES

1.1.1 Application

Until recently the Centralized Hospital Eye Service Appointment Scheme (CHESAS) organized HES pre-registration positions but this has now been replaced by a company called JCL Consulting and further information can be found at http://www.jclconsulting.co.uk. The application forms for this scheme must be filled in and returned by the closing date along with a small fee. JCL will forward the applications to the hospital optometry departments and then correspondence from each department will be directly with you. There is no point in applying to those hospitals that participate in CHESAS in any other way. However, not all hospital optometry departments take part in the scheme; other hospitals should be applied to directly. If you are very keen on spending your pre-registration year in the HES then it is best to apply to every hospital optometry department as early as you can.

1.1.2 Advantages

Advantages of spending the pre-registration year in the HES include:

- You will be working as part of a team, often with other hospital pre-registration optometrists or visiting pre-registration optometrists from primary care optometric practices
- You do not need to concern yourself with too many commercial constraints of optometric practice and often will not have to balance concerns about the cost of the optometric care required with the ability of the patient to pay
- You will be exposed to a wide range of abnormal ocular conditions. You will have a chance to examine many post-cataract, keratoconus, low-vision, and other patients who present infrequently in primary care optometric practice
- You may gain substantial experience in paediatric optometry, low vision, ultrasound and the use of drugs in optometric practice
- You will have easy access to ophthalmology and orthoptic clinics and may be able to take part in specialized contact lens fitting and low vision clinics
- Experience of hospital practice will be useful for your career. Specialized experience will come in useful if you work in primary care optometric practice in the future and you will be in a good position to inform patients what will happen to them if you need to refer them to the HES
- The professional staff in the hospital will be invaluable for answering any questions that may arise during your work or revision. Ophthalmologists and optometrists at the hospital might even be coexaminers
- You are likely to have access to a full range of optometric equipment, some of which might not be available in a primary care optometric practice
- With day or block placements in primary care optometric practice and possibly other external visits (e.g. factory tours), you will be able to experience the full range of optometric procedures
- You will probably get Saturdays off!

1.1.3 Disadvantages

It is possible that there may not be any day or block placements in primary care optometric practice and you may miss out on the experience of commercial considerations and aspects of practice; these are very likely to be of use in your career.

You may not see very much in the way of 'normal' patients. A high percentage of your refractions may be on patients with ocular pathology. You may not have much chance to practise your full eye examination routine. The day-to-day work of the clinic might involve providing refraction results for ophthalmologists who will not require you to perform binocular investigations, ophthalmoscopy or slit lamp examination. Of course you may be able to find time to practise these skills anyway and it is important for the Routine PQE that you are practised in performing a comprehensive eye examination routine within the imposed time limit.

It might be difficult to follow a full eye examination on a patient with dispensing. This is important for the case records you will need to submit, and for the Dispensing PQE.

These disadvantages can be overcome by spending time away from the hospital in primary care optometric practice. However, your hospital employer might not allow you time off to do this and you may have to sacrifice your Saturdays off!

1.1.4 Comments from employers

When interviewing a candidate, employers say they look for:

- Candidates who are keen, intelligent, neat, polite, and articulate, showing enthusiasm for and commitment to optometry, with a particular interest in hospital work. They should be willing to learn, able to communicate and explain a variety of topics, show initiative and have sought to improve their experience already. 'We are looking for someone who will work well in a multidisciplinary environment.'
- A sense of humour and the ability not to take one's self too seriously are advantages! The common sense essential for good clinical judgement and a genuine interest in people that leads ultimately to becoming a caring professional are important

Hospital employers say this about the advantages of a pre-registration year in hospital:

- The experience of hospital supervisors makes them good teachers with a good knowledge of the standards required to pass the PQEs
- The continuous process of multi-disciplinary teaching programmes
- The broadest possible range of experience and a wide variety of patients

not available in primary care practice, but the chance to work in primary care practice one day a week
- Access to external courses and study leave
- Development of communication skills through seeing a wide variety of patients
- Often hospital accommodation is available and hence the potential for an active social life!
- The wide experience of abnormal ocular conditions and opportunities to attend tutorials and visits in other departments of the hospital
- The benefits of being in a team environment – both social and educational
- The advantages of meetings and discussions with a wide variety of eye care professionals.

Their expectations of a pre-registration optometrist are:

- To be prepared to work hard and to take an interest in the problems and welfare of their patients
- To take advantage of the teaching opportunities available to them – including teaching sessions out of working hours, use of the medical library, etc.
- To be courteous to patients and staff
- A transition from a trainee who needs to be checked at each step into an active junior member of the team
- Good attitude to hard work and learning appreciated.

Other comments for pre-registration optometrists and final year students:

- Optometry can be a very lucrative profession. New optometrists are urged not to make finance their main priority in the first few years, but instead to make sure that they have the best possible grounding from which to make future choices
- Experiences missed, including a spell in hospital optometry are very difficult to make up later
- It's good to get work experience in holidays and on Saturdays, whether optical or not. This gives practice at hard work, dealing with public and colleagues, and timekeeping etc. It is then less of a shock when you begin the arduous pre-registration year. This includes daily 'nine to five' work in clinics plus revising in the evenings.

1.2 INDEPENDENT PRACTICE

1.2.1 Application

Application for pre-registration positions in an independent practice is normally by direct correspondence with the proprietor or manager of the practice. A list of approved supervisors and practices is enclosed in a CO second year mailing. You may wish to contact all the approved practices in the area where you would like to work. When contacting practices in your chosen area, enclose a cover letter and a concise CV. Again, we strongly advise you to contact your university careers centre for support in developing and preparing your CV and cover letter. Remember each year there are more people seeking pre-registration placements than there are positions available, so anything that makes your application stand out from the rest (in a positive way) can only help your cause. Practices seeking applications will sometimes advertise in the professional press or contact the universities; advertisements for positions may appear on departmental notice boards. Check these boards every day and apply immediately you see a placement that seems to meet your requirements.

1.2.2 Advantages

You may be given much more freedom in an independent practice. You have a direct relationship with the owner or manager, and this should allow for efficient management of your requirements. If you need time off for a factory visit or revision, it is likely that your supervisor will be able to ensure that it is allowed.

Independent practices allow you to shape your own pre-registration year, without being sent on courses or dragged to presentations or tutorials that you may feel are of little use. You can manage your own time and arrange your own courses and activities with help and support from your supervisor and practice. Often (but not always), your employer will pay for courses and examination fees.

Normally, if working in an independent practice, arrangements will be made for you to attend a hospital eye department at least one day per week. However you may be expected to arrange block release at the local hospital, possibly doing a swap with the hospital pre-registration optometrist and visit the hospital every day for one or two weeks during the year.

1.2.3 Disadvantages

- In an independent practice, you may not have access to the variety of experience that can be provided in hospital practice
- You may not be given a structured programme of training and assessment as might be provided when working for a multiple
- It is unlikely that you will be working in a large team of professionals as in hospital practice, and therefore you will be unable to confer with other pre-registration optometrists to the same extent that you could in a multiple company or hospital practice where it is likely that several pre-registration optometrists will be employed

- It may not be possible to obtain supplementary optometric equipment as easily as in hospital or multiple practice.

1.2.4 Comments from employers

When interviewing a candidate, employers say that:

- Presentation, smart appearance, a quiet confident manner, good speech – 'should be able to speak the King's English' (sic), and friendliness are important. Enthusiasm about optometry and evidence of interest around the subject, and good communication skills.

Employers say the advantages of a pre-registration year in independent practice are:

- Experience with a wide range of patients
- Access to hospital experience
- Examination fees paid (sometimes)
- Supervisor may be a CO examiner
- Arrangements for evening tutorials
- Pre-registration optometrists are encouraged to develop clinical and patient management skills
- Personal supervision by experienced optometrists
- Fully equipped consulting room and opportunities for workshop and glazing experience
- Time is allowed for pre-examination study and refresher courses.

These comments are taken from several employers and indicate their opinions of the advantages of a pre-registration year with them. Obviously, certain provisions will be specific to individual appointments. However, the list gives an idea of the types of advantage that independent employers consider important.

Their expectations of a pre-registration optometrist are:

- A commitment to developing skills after passing the PQEs – just because you have qualified doesn't mean you have mastered the job
- Not to rush home at 5pm on the dot
- Conscientious and diligent eye examination, attention to detail
- Ability to do small repairs and adjustments, fitting spectacles to patients and dispensing
- Enthusiasm and willingness to learn and to work hard.

Other comments for pre-registration optometrist and final-year students:

- Keep reading journals and textbooks
- Look up everything you're not sure about and ask questions. You will only get out what you put in

- Rely on your own ability with hand instruments rather than auto-refractors; competent retinoscopy is far more reliable and in many cases essential

1.3 MULTIPLE PRACTICE

1.3.1 Application

Application for a pre-registration position with a supervisor in a practice that belongs to a corporate body is made to the head office of the company. The second year mailing from the CO contains addresses of several companies along with the names of the people responsible for recruitment. Normally you should write (probably best to enclose a stamped addressed envelope) requesting an application form. Application forms will usually require you to provide details of qualifications and work experience (and possibly a current CV) and your preferences for particular locations. University careers officers will be glad to offer support in completing these forms. There will often be a series of interviews, possibly at head office or in a venue near your university, and then probably another at the practice. It is imperative that you meet your prospective supervisor and visit your proposed practice before agreeing to take the position.

1.3.2 Advantages

- Multiples have a reputation for providing good structured training programmes, including in-house courses and continuous assessment. Different companies structure their pre-registration year in various ways. Often courses and tutorials will provide an opportunity for you to meet fellow pre-registration optometrists and discuss aspects of your progress
- Multiples may be able to give you experience of working in several different practices. This is useful to encourage the flexibility required in the examinations, where you will be expected to perform competently in an unfamiliar environment
- A large company may have a team of training personnel, usually optometrists who are often examiners. The team will have experience in training pre-registration optometrists and dealing with problems commonly encountered. They will also be experienced at assessing candidates and well-qualified to give constructive advice. Some multiples will arrange for you to take mock PQEs, providing useful experience before the actual examinations
- Multiples are well organized in arranging hospital experience and time off for educational visits during the pre-registration year
- Often your employer will pay for courses and exam fees.

1.3.3 Disadvantages

- Multiples may not be able to provide the one-to-one attention and personal guidance that could be given in an independent practice
- A pre-registration year with a multiple may not provide the wide range of experience in ophthalmology and related fields that can be gained in the HES
- You may prefer to choose and arrange your own courses and activities during the year, rather than be expected to attend those arranged for you by the company. The company might expect you to attend its own courses rather than external ones, which you may feel, would be more useful. You may be expected to take annual leave in order to go on external courses.

1.3.4 Comments from employers

When interviewing a candidate, employers say:

- We look for students who appear to best possess the personal skills they feel are necessary for a pre-registration optometrist. Application forms (or CVs) presented in a neat and logical manner are more likely to be selected.
- Important attributes include: smart appearance, good educational record, good capacity for clinical reasoning, any relevant work experience (not necessarily optical), good communication skills, ability to work well in a team environment, pleasant personality, out-going, adaptable, ambition and self-discipline, awareness of current professional and commercial matters, good organizational and decision-making skills.
- Lively personality (but not too lively!). Genuine interest in people. Enthusiastic all-rounder, good communication skills, enjoyment of the clinical side of the job. Interest in a career with the company. Clear understanding of the optometrist's role and good communication skills. Ability to work as part of the practice team.

Advantages of a pre-registration year in a multiple company:

- Well-structured pre-registration year with support and experience provided
- The trainee/supervisor pair are allocated an experienced tutor
- Each trainee receives a pre-registration manual containing useful information about the year (sometimes!)
- Manuals contain subject information and exercises that are marked by tutors
- Central courses containing mock exams
- Personal study programme – feedback on written work, group discussion and seminars

- Hospital experience. Student loan service (sometimes)
- Students allowed to attend external courses
- Busy, well-equipped practices with a good range of patients to examine
- Trained supervisors
- Experience of different practices/supervisors
- Examination fees paid.

Their expectations of the pre-registration optometrist are:

- It is hoped that the trainee will enjoy the year with the company and wish to continue working for it after qualifying. The trainee is expected to give their best at all times during the year. There are expectations on numbers of eye examinations completed, other than those required by the CO.
- To have shaken off 'the student mentality', and to adopt a responsible attitude and helpful approach to patients. To attend all courses and opportunities made available. The trainees have to fit in to the working environment and to initially work at their own speed, building confidence and eventually helping with the workload of the practice. After three months the trainee is expected to be examining around eight to ten patients per day (check with your employer).

Other comments for pre-registration optometrists and final-year students:

- Be as pro-active as possible in your training during the year, in other words make the most of what is offered and do not sit back and wait for things to happen, because they probably won't
- Final year students should prepare for interviews and arrive looking the part
- Complete all application forms with extreme care
- Remember you are in competition with everyone else
- Be honest with yourself and any future employer
- Apply at the end of the second year or early at the beginning of the final year (it's worth it for the peace of mind of having secured a position)
- Evidence of work experience, preferably in an optometry practice or working with the public (restaurants, shops) is desirable.

1.4 THE INTERVIEW

When one of us (MH) was interviewed for his pre-registration position, the supervisor thought she was assessing him as a prospective trainee. He had other ideas. After it had been established that he was a relatively pleasant and intelligent young man (*sic*), he produced a long list of questions he wanted answered to ensure he would be looked after during his pre-registration year. This seemed to astonish but at the same time impress the supervisor and he got the job! The interview is an opportunity for your prospective employer to assess your suitability and for you to ensure that the position offered is the right one for you.

It is imperative that you meet your prospective supervisor at the time of the interview, or at least at some point before you sign your contract of employment. This is the person with whom you will be working on a one-to-one basis throughout your pre-registration year. Your supervisor will guide your clinical decision-making, advise you, and monitor your work, particularly your case records. It can also be helpful to meet optometrists who spent their pre-registration year with the practice/supervisor. Ask questions during the interview and satisfy yourself that the supervisor or employer can guarantee you the best possible opportunity to prepare for the PQEs. Do not be intimidated at the interview and feel that asking for points to be clarified or making requests for certain 'extras' within your pre-registration year will be frowned upon. It is important to make clear your needs and expectations for the year and be satisfied that your prospective employer will be able to fulfil these requirements.

Do not place any importance on the size of the salary offered. Most employers will base this on the recommended NHS rate. It is not worth looking for a slightly better package at the expense of good training. If you have to take re-sits and delay qualification it will cost you more financially than you would gain from having a slightly higher pre-registration salary.

1.4.1 Questions you may like to ask at the interview

1 How many eye examinations (it is better to use this phrase rather than sight tests, especially when talking with independent optometrists) will I be expected to carry out daily:
   (a) In the first month?
   (b) In subsequent months?
   (c) In the weeks leading up to the examinations?
2 What provision will be made for hospital/primary care practice experience?
3 What period of revision leave will I be allowed prior to each set of examinations?
4 What provision will be made for attendance at revision courses prior to the examinations – in-house/external?
5 Will I be able to choose which courses I attend throughout the year? Will the employer fund these?
6 Will my examination fees be paid?
7 Are there prospects for my future employment at the end of the year:
   (a) If I qualify?
   (b) If I have to re-sit?
8 Will re-sit fees be paid?

9 Will time be put aside on a regular basis for discussion of cases and problems arising within the pre-registration year? How often?

10 How much time will be set aside for discussion and preparation of my case records? How many people will be available to look through these case records?

11 Apart from holidays/illness, will my supervisor be in regular attendance? Will I have more than one supervisor?

12 What support staff does the practice have?

13 Will I have my own *fully equipped* consulting room?

14 What equipment will be at my disposal? (See Section 1.4.2)

15 If certain equipment is not currently available, will it be provided?

16 What provision will be made for the fitting of contact lenses? What types of contact lenses are fitted within the practice?

17 Is there scope for fitting different types of contact lenses other than those already used in the practice?

18 Will there be an opportunity to undertake supervised domiciliary work?

19 Will provision be made for experience in specialist fields:
   (a) Low vision?
   (b) Contact lens work?
   (c) Orthoptics?
   (d) Industrial optics – safety/lighting?
   (e) Manufacturing optics?

20 What will be the hours of employment?

21 How many weeks holiday will I get?

22 Will I need to use annual leave to attend courses?

23 What will my salary be?

24 When will I be expected to start?

Some of these issues may be dealt with earlier in the interview and you may think of others; this list is a guide to the sort of things you will need to know. Take a pen and paper with you to take down notes. You will normally be shown the practice(s) in which you might be working; if not, it is important that you arrange a visit before signing a contract.

1.4.2 Equipment list

You should check that you will be provided with all the equipment you require during the pre-registration year, or at least be sure that special equipment can be loaned to you from other sources when required. The following list suggests the basic requirements that you should expect to have easy access to.

1 Basic eye examination equipment – specify your preferences for illuminated/projector chart, trial case/phoropter, and your requirements for trial frame, retinoscope, ophthalmoscope, crossed cylinders and confirmation lenses if you do not possess your own.

  2 Amsler charts
  3 Colour vision tests
  4 Tonometer – contact/non-contact
  5 Visual field screener
  6 Fixation disparity tests
  7 Maddox rod, Maddox wing, RAF rule, near vision chart
  8 Slit lamp biomicroscope
  9 Condensing lenses
10 Keratometer
11 Focimeter
12 Burton lamp
13 Inter-pupillary distance gauge
14 Stereopsis test(s)
15 Drugs:
    (a) cycloplegics
    (b) mydriatics
    (c) diagnostics
    (d) topical anaesthetics
    (e) anti-infectives
16 Children's vision tests
17 Prism bars
18 Text books
19 *Optician* and *OT* journals.

2

Pre-registration year calendar

This chapter is intended to be a guide, highlighting what to do before starting your pre-registration year, how to approach the year and finishing with successful completion of your examinations. We have included details of mailings you will receive from the CO and action to be taken at various points throughout the year.

UNIVERSITY FINAL YEAR

Spring term

A CO mailing will be sent to you and will include:

- A covering letter containing advice about making arrangements for your pre-registration year.
- Details of the CHESAS
- A copy of the CO pre-registration training pack including:
  - Enrolment in the pre-registration year
  - A guide on steps to registration
  - Syllabus and regulations for the PQEs Part II
  - Appraisals
- CD-ROM containing:
  - PQE Part II work sheets
  - Recommended reading
  - Adverts for refresher courses
  - Code of Ethics and Guidance for Professional Conduct
  - Optometrists Formulary
  - Supplementary sources of information.

We very strongly advise you to read every word of this information, and when you have finished, read it again! It is advisable at this time to begin applying for a pre-registration position, see Chapter 1. Enrolment form PR1 is particularly important and should be completed when you obtain your degree result and returned to the CO to start the pre-registration year enrolment procedure. Now, concentrate on your final year university examinations. Good luck!

Summer term

Immediately upon receiving your degree result, enrol for the pre-registration year by submitting form PR1 to the CO (plus enrolment fee). Note, there are sections on this form for both the pre-registration trainee and the supervisor to complete, and the pre-registration year will not officially start until the completed form has been received and processed by the CO. For those who have not been offered a pre-registration position and are therefore unable to meet the deadline, PR1 forms should be submitted as soon as an offer is made. It is important not to leave it too late to submit form PR1, as you need to have at least 12 months experience before becoming eligible for registration. You will not be able to register without 12 months experience even if you have passed all your PQEs. If you do not receive confirmation of receipt of form PR1 within four weeks of sending it, then contact the CO.

In acknowledgement of receiving form PR1 and the enrolment fee, the CO will send you a letter confirming the official start date of your pre-registration year. Now take a short break or holiday! You probably need it and definitely deserve it.

THE PRE-REGISTRATION YEAR

Summer

During your first week in practice, get used to the surroundings, facilities and general organization before thinking about starting to perform eye examinations. Make notes of any special requirements you have or extra equipment you need and talk to your supervisor about these.

Autumn

During September/October the CO will send an EX1 examination application form. It is advisable to submit the examination entry form as soon as possible in order to have the best chance of being accepted to sit the examinations at your preferred centre. This may be particularly important to you if one of the examination centres happens to be at the university you attended. We strongly advise you to send the completed examination entry form back to the CO on the same day you receive it and use first-class post. This will give you a very good chance, of being examined at the centre of your choice since places are allocated on a first come, first served basis. You do not have to send payment with the application, but the CO must receive payment by the closing date of entry.

Take note of the closing dates for submission of case records. Keep a logbook listing names of every patient you see, along with brief notes on the nature of your results. This will be useful when choosing case records to write up for submission.

Make sure you have a comprehensive plan of action for the period from now until March, when you may be sitting the first set of examinations. Plan the following:

- Meetings with other pre-registration optometrists in your area to discuss aspects of your training
- Refresher courses and tutorials
- Local optical society meetings (these are often free for pre-registration optometrists)
- Provision of experience in the HES and primary care practice as appropriate. This should already have been arranged by now
- Visits to orthoptic clinics, low vision clinics, manufacturing opticians, industrial plants (in relation to safety and lighting for the Occupational optometry PQE).

To help make your plans see Chapter 4; Making the most of your pre-registration year and refresher courses.

If you are not sitting the exams at a venue with which you are familiar, you may like to attend a course at the venue, or simply contact the clinic manager and arrange a visit so that you can familiarize yourself with the layout.

Start to prepare a few case records now and show them to your supervisor. The preparation of case records is a very lengthy process and involves many failed attempts and revisions before your reports are perfected.

Your three-month review form should be completed about this time, in conjunction with your supervisor, and submitted to your nominated adviser or to the College if you do not have an adviser.

You should receive confirmation of your examination entry any time now.

December

Make sure your arrangements for the PQEs have been confirmed and that you have sent the required fee to the CO by the closing date. You should have drafted a significant proportion of your case records by now. If you have not arranged to attend any courses and you wish to do so, then do it now. Also, now is the time to arrange your accommodation at the examination centre – see Chapter 5 for details.

January to March

Plan your revision and revise for the first set of examinations. Give a complete draft set of case records to your supervisor for review. You will receive your individual examination timetable approximately one month before your examinations are due to start.

March

Your six-month review form should be completed about this time, in conjunction with your supervisor, and submitted to your nominated adviser or to the CO if you do not have an adviser.

March to May

First set of PQEs

This covers anomalies of binocular vision, use of drugs in optometric practice, investigative techniques, partial sight and its management, occupational optometry, and dispensing (not necessarily in this order). You won't receive your results until after you have taken the second set of PQEs in June or July.

Complete final copies of the case records. At least four weeks before the closing date for submission and make sure that you give your supervisor your final draft for review. Ask other optometrists you know to look at them and make comments. No matter how perfect you think they are, there will be mistakes to correct. *Submit your case records before the closing date and keep a copy.*

June to July

Second set of PQEs

This covers routine examination, case records and law, ocular disease and abnormality, contact lenses (not necessarily in this order), followed by the assessment board.

Following the second set of PQEs, you will be advised of your results for both sets at the assessment board. If some of your results are 'borderline' you may be examined again during the assessment board. This involves a viva, with one or more examiners asking questions on those topics that you just failed in the exams, before your final result is decided. There will be little time if any to prepare for this.

If you are successful, you will be sent the following:

- Registration papers for the General Optical Council (GOC)
- Application for membership of the CO.

Well done!

On completion of your required period of supervised clinical training (normally 12 months) you must submit form M2A to the CO confirming that you have carried out the specified number of refractions, dispensing and contact lens fits, and aftercares.

If you have failed any examinations, one of the assessment board members will inform you which ones you will need to re-sit. Don't worry, you are in the majority! See Chapter 6 – Re-takes.

September

Re-takes may be at any of the university departments; the CO will inform you of the venue options. You will be asked to re-sit only the subjects that you failed earlier in the year.

December

Re-takes are at the Institute of Optometry in London only. You will be expected to re-sit the subjects that you failed in September. Following the December re-takes, if you still have not passed all ten examinations you will be required to wait at least 12 months before sitting all ten PQEs again! Unfortunately more and more candidates are finding themselves in this position. However, it is still possible to pass next time round!

3

The College of Optometrists and the examiners

The CO organizes the PQEs on behalf of the GOC in order to ensure that trainees have enough practical experience prior to registration. From the end of the second year at university, the CO will be in contact with you and guide you through finding a pre-registration position, taking the examinations and eventually to registration. If you have a query about any aspect of the pre-registration year, the CO should be able to help you or refer you to somebody who can.

The examiners are recruited and trained by the CO. Most examiners are optometrists, but there may be a lighting engineer examining in the occupational optometry PQE and an ophthalmologist in the ocular disease and abnormality PQE.

This book has been written independently and does not represent the views of the CO. However, we would like to acknowledge the valuable help and advice that we received from the CO. The remainder of this chapter consists of answers to questions we asked of a former PQE co-ordinator.

3.1 WHAT TRAINING DO EXAMINERS RECEIVE?

'The CO recruits examiners from time to time by advertisement. Prospective examiners must have at least four years post-qualification experience, show evidence of continuing education and be sponsored by two CO members. Prior to commencing as examiners they must attend an induction programme that deals with the examination format, examination techniques and the aims of the PQEs. As part of this training they undergo specific interview skills training using role-play and video playback on an individual basis.

On the first occasion on which they examine, probationary (new) examiners will sit in with two experienced examiners and observe for one day and then actively examine on the second day. One of the experienced examiners will act as moderator. On all occasions, the experienced examiners will write a report on the probationary examiner's performance. These are monitored and those showing no adverse examining problems are confirmed in post after the first year. Examiners who show some difficulties will be asked to continue for a second probationary year after which they will be asked to stand down or will be confirmed in post, depending on performance. All existing examiners have undergone this training.

Examiners' meetings are held on a regular basis either by section or as a meeting of all examiners. At the large meetings, examiners will hear presentations on examination techniques used by other medical, paramedical and certification bodies.

Roving examiners who monitor examiner consistency and form the basis of the assessment boards have undergone further training on appraisal interview skills so that they can offer constructive advice to examiners on any poor examining practices that they may come across.

All examiner appointments are subject to review after five years.'

3.2 WHAT CRITICISMS DO YOU HAVE OF THE PRESENT PQE SYSTEM?

'The present examination format was inherited by the CO from the founding bodies. Since that time, numerous refinements have been made. Examiner audit in the form of roving examiners has also been introduced to assist the consistency of the PQEs. However, it must be accepted that with between 500 and 650 candidates being examined in ten sections at several examination centres and with over 120 examiners, consistency is an ongoing concern.

The CO has the dual duty of ensuring fair examination while maintaining the public duty of preventing anyone not fit to practice from gaining entry to the register.'

3.3 WHAT CHANGES ARE PLANNED FOR THE PQEs IN THE FUTURE?

'The CO liaises with examiners on a continuing basis and suggestions are often made for the improvement of the examination. There are no plans for further refinements of the existing examination at present.' (*At the time of the interview the CO did not have any plans to change the PQEs, but recently a new format has been considered – see the Introduction, p. ix.*)

3.4 DO YOU HAVE ANY ADVICE FOR FIRST-TIME CANDIDATES/CANDIDATES TAKING RE-SITS?

'The main advice to candidates taking for the first time is to remember that oral examinations require a more structured thinking process. The breadth and complexity of the syllabus does not permit learning by rote. The requirement is to be able to use the existing knowledge to work out answers to clinical problems that might not have been experienced before. For this reason it is important to have a good grasp of fundamental subjects such as anatomy and physiology, which might have been learned early in a university course but which are of fundamental importance to the understanding of clinical problems.

Re-take candidates must accept responsibility for their failure and look as objectively as possible at their own performance. Examiners' comments found on the failure report and the examination department staff (at the CO) can offer guidance as required.'

3.5 WHAT IS THE RELATIONSHIP BETWEEN THE GOC AND THE CO AS FAR AS THE PQEs ARE CONCERNED?

'The GOC is responsible for ensuring that those applying for registration meet the necessary standards to practice safely. The GOC recognizes the CO examination as fulfilling that function in conjunction with a pre-registration year when a required number of eye examinations and dispensings have been undertaken under supervision.

As a "delegated function", the GOC visits the CO examinations on a five-year cycle to confirm that the standards being applied are appropriate and that the exam is fair and relevant. While the CO is at liberty to change the examination as it sees fit, inappropriate, substantial change might cause the GOC to review its approval of the examination as a means of gaining registration.'

3.6 RUMOURS

We also asked the former co-ordinator to comment on certain rumours about the PQEs that had come to light during our research for this book. We have chosen simply to print the responses, which will hopefully put an end to some misconceptions people have about the PQEs.

'Luck' in the exams

'All examinations, since they cannot assess the whole syllabus, must involve an element of chance. If you are asked a question that you know and the next candidate is asked a question which he or she does not know, this could be construed as luck. Nevertheless, the examination is a sampling procedure and the candidate will generally only fail if there is inadequacy over a range of areas. The exception to this might be failure to detect obvious pathology in an examination, which could have serious implications. This could, in itself, cause failure. Standards are monitored by roving examiners and are moderated by the assessment board, which has powers to re-assess candidates in cases of doubt.'

Objectivity of examiners

'Lack of objectivity (among examiners) rarely arises, since every attempt is made (as far as the constraints of the timetable allow) for candidates not to be assessed by the same examiner during the main examinations or in the same subject at re-sits. They would certainly not be re-examined by the same pair of examiners. The training already in place deals with these issues. Candidates are probably unaware of the amount of training undertaken by examiners or the amount of monitoring that occurs.'

Standards

'Standards (for passing examinations) are laid down in the guidelines and do not vary. The section pass rate (percentage of candidates passing) has averaged between 70 and 90 per cent (depending on the section). Given this pass rate across ten sections, it is a simple mathematical calculation to determine the probability of passing all ten sections at one sitting. There is no influence involved from the CO but it is a function of the examination format.

Since the PQE account runs on a break-even basis, there is no financial gain (for the CO) from having anyone re-sit the examination. Indeed, it might be a more logical argument to propose that the CO has a vested interest in getting membership fees at the earliest opportunity!'

Appeal procedures

'To successfully appeal against the examiners' decision it must be shown that the examination has not been conducted according to the regulations or that there was a serious failure in the assessment procedure. Unfortunately most appeals are based on the candidate disagreeing with the verdict of the examiners. Successful appeals have been made where they are justified and have resulted in early re-examination or re-assessment.'

Counselling provided following exam failure

'The counselling procedure is designed to isolate areas of preparation that could be improved or areas of clinical experience that need expanding. In some cases significant amounts of time are spent in encouraging the candidates to accept responsibility for their own failure rather than blaming colleagues, supervisors or examiners. As with all counselling, if the candidate will not accept the reality of the situation, help cannot be given. By definition, counselling helps candidates determine their own solutions; it is not provided to tell them how to pass the examination, which is what many actually would prefer. In such a wide-ranging examination, sound and wide-ranging preparation is the only way to pass.'

Problems faced by overseas candidates

'It is clear that in a viva examination where verbal communication is the means of indicating knowledge and skill, a reasonable working knowledge of the English language and optometric vocabulary is required. Examiners' comments indicate that where there is apparent language difficulty, the main problem is getting sufficient answers to make a judgement on competence in the time available.

In the preliminary examination for non-UK and non-EC candidates, the CO has moved away from essay-style questions and onto multiple-choice questions to ease the language problem. This examination is equivalent to optometry degree level and successful candidates will still need to sit the Part 2 PQEs.'

3.7 OUR ADVICE

It is clear that a great deal of care is taken to ensure consistency and fairness when assessing candidates. However, if you think you were treated unfairly in an examination, keep a record of exactly why you think this and what led to it. Inform a member of the CO examinations staff as soon as possible, preferably immediately after the examination. It may be too late to complain after you have received your results. If you have any questions about the examinations, or would like information about counselling and support for failed sections, then contact the CO.

4

Making the most of the pre-registration year and refresher courses

The pre-registration year is not only about preparing for the examinations. It is also about putting theory into practice, mastering the patient and practitioner relationship, mastering your equipment, learning how to prevent things from going wrong and what to do when things do go wrong (e.g. non-tolerance cases), and the development of new skills (e.g. domiciliary examinations). To be properly prepared for the PQEs involves all of these things. The experience gained from a varied pre-registration year will show in your examinations. You will not be spoon-fed during the pre-registration year and must work hard with your supervisor to make sure that you achieve all that you should.

This chapter has two parts. The first part deals with how to make the most of your pre-registration year irrespective of the type of practice you work in. The second part highlights courses that are available for the pre-registration optometrist.

4.1 MAKING THE MOST OF THE PRE-REGISTRATION YEAR

There are four areas of optometry in which a PQE candidate can work during their pre-registration year: multiple practice; independent practice; university practice; and hospital practice. Of course, there is no such thing as the ideal pre-registration position and all of these options have disadvantages as well as advantages (these have been described in Chapter 1). However, it may take several weeks before the disadvantages become apparent, by which time it may be too late to do anything about them. The aim of this section is to highlight the advantages and disadvantages, with suggestions as to how to make the most of the former and to overcome the latter.

4.1.1 General points

The following general points apply to all types of pre-registration positions.

In order to make the most of the pre-registration year, trainees should, in conjunction with their supervisors, produce a plan for the year even before it starts. This book will be a useful aid in drawing up this plan (see Chapter 2). The pre-registration year usually begins in August and the first set of six examinations is usually in March or April. This leaves eight to nine months in which to cover six topics in detail, as well as keeping up on the other four subjects. A detailed plan or timetable is necessary to prevent leaving topics until the last minute. This goes especially for case studies. Make a note of any interesting cases you see that may be used for case records. Be prepared to hand in to your supervisor, at least in draft format, three case records every month, and then write up properly when they are satisfactory.

As well as having responsibility for a pre-registration optometrist, your supervisor will also be expected to carry out a full day's work, examining patients and probably have some involvement in the day-to-day management of the practice. Supervisors are busy people and sometimes you may not be their top priority. Ask your supervisor to sit in with you as often as possible, at least once a week, and watch you carry out a full routine examination, fit contact lenses, carry out aftercares and apply investigative techniques. Encourage your supervisor to make notes, to ask questions at the end, and follow up with a critical analysis of your techniques with pointers on how to improve them. This should become a more frequent event after the December holidays and will result in you becoming used to being observed while examining patients. Practical PQEs are likely to be more traumatic for trainees not used to a third party observing them as they work. Closer to the examinations your supervisor should set aside time to conduct mock oral exams on as many of the examination subjects as possible. Again, critical analysis at the end of each session is imperative. If possible you should make use of a camcorder to video your performance and carry out a self-analysis. This may highlight some personal habits that an examiner might find tiresome.

If you spend your year in an area with a nearby university optometry department, apply to join the university library. A fee will be charged, but this will be more than offset by access to optometry journals and textbooks, as well as providing a quiet place to study. Local non-optometric libraries can also arrange interlibrary loans of articles and textbooks. It is strongly recommended that you subscribe to the *Optician* magazine, which along with *OT* (*Optometry Today* – this is free) have excellent articles on contact lenses, spectacle lenses, pathology, low vision aids, and law, as well as giving the trainee a feel for general developments in optometry.

4.1.2 The pre-registration year in multiple, independent and university practice

The pre-registration year is broadly similar in these three environments as far as clinical advantages and disadvantages are concerned so they will be covered together.

Working in primary care (i.e. non-hospital) practice has the clinical advantage of regular full routine eye examinations. However, there is a danger that this will be all that the trainee will be allowed to do. Early in the year discuss with your supervisor how many contact lens patients you will see each week for new fits and how many for aftercares. Ask to do dispensing, visual field analyses and VDU screenings if your practice has this facility.

The main disadvantage of primary care practice is the low number of pathology and binocular vision cases that present. Ask your supervisor to let you examine any pathology or binocular vision cases they come across. Most general practices have an arrangement for their trainees to visit the HES, for which the hospital will receive a payment. These visits may involve a half or whole day in hospital per week and are (in theory) designed to give the trainee personal one-to-one tuition with an ophthalmologist, while on duty in the eye casualty department or in the outpatient department, or with an orthoptist. Your supervisor will probably liaise directly with the hospital's head optometrist (if there is one) and this will be your main contact. You should ask to spend at least half the day with the ophthalmologist for pathology experience, or half with the orthoptist for binocular vision experience, once a week. If this does not happen report to your supervisor. Remember your training within the HES has been paid for!

While at the hospital make contact with some of the junior ophthalmologists. As part of their training they are required to pass an examination in refraction and no matter how inexperienced you feel as a pre-registration optometrist, you will have infinitely more knowledge on refraction than a junior ophthalmologist. Arrangements can be made whereby you 'sit in' with a junior ophthalmologist in eye casualty (probably outside normal working hours), in return for refraction tuition, perhaps using the hospital optometry department facilities.

4.1.3 Hospital practice

The great advantage of a year in hospital practice is that there is a great deal of pathology and large numbers of patients with binocular vision anomalies. There should be regular timetabled sessions for the trainee to observe in casualty, the outpatient department or in the orthoptic department. It is important to seek permission first from your supervisor (usually the head of the optometry department) and then from the consultant ophthalmologist or head orthoptist. Quiet moments in the optometry department (very rare) can be made use of by spending extra time in these clinics. You should endeavour to 'sit in' all the specialist clinics, e.g. diabetes, glaucoma and retina, as often as your work schedule allows. Befriending a junior ophthalmologist may allow extra sessions in casualty outside work hours in return for refraction tuition.

The main disadvantage of a pre-registration year in the HES is the lack of full routine eye examination opportunities. Some can be arranged on hospital workers, but this usually has to be done outside normal working hours. Standard hospital refraction usually consists of retinoscopy and subjective refraction. Keen trainees may conduct ophthalmoscopy remembering that they are not allowed to write their results in the patient's notes, but the heavy workload rarely allows this to be done on a regular basis. Most hospital optometry departments have primary care optometrists who attend on a sessional basis for half or one day per week. These can be approached to arrange occasional sessions in private practice for full routine examinations on 'normal' patients. The supervisor can also be approached for assistance with such a placement, as lack of full routine patients is a well-recognized problem in hospital training and such a release scheme may already exist. Two of us (FE and MMR) spent our pre-registration year in the HES, where we gained invaluable experience and knowledge and have no regrets about our choice.

For those working in Greater London, the Institute of Optometry organizes evening clinics for pre-registration optometrists. The clinics involve general refraction, binocular vision, contact lenses, and investigative techniques. There is a charge to the trainee. Clinics begin in the autumn and continue to the summer. They provide a wide variety of patients that may not be met in primary care practice and an opportunity for those in hospital practice to develop their full routine skills. Supervisors, some of whom are also examiners, staff the clinics. There are also tutorials and evening lectures aimed at preparation for the PQEs.

4.1.4 Study groups

Problems that may seem insurmountable to you as an individual often seem less so when approached by a group. This is true for the PQEs. By forming a study group, which may vary in size from around two to ten or more, the pre-registration year and the PQEs can be tackled more efficiently. Such a group can be formed reasonably easily. You may know of other trainees who are working in your area. Your supervisor may know of other supervisors with trainees. Phone round local practices and ask if there is a trainee. Pre-registration optometrists working for the same multiple may meet at company functions. Fellow trainees can be found via attendance at local optical society meetings. The CO may even help you find other local trainees These contacts are best made in the first two to three weeks of the year and meetings arranged at least on a monthly basis. We don't consider the pub to be a good venue!

Although some trainees prefer not to share information and keep hold of those obscure but important details gleaned from a journal or their supervisor, trainees are not competing among themselves but are 'competing against' the examiners. Question and answer sessions are a useful way of sorting out problems. Information is easier to remember after it has been discussed rather than just read. You will have spent three or more years writing about optometry and probably do this very well. However the PQEs are mostly about verbal communication and this is something that has to be practised. Verbal discussion will reveal how well you know and understand a topic.

Your group could invite lecturers from the nearest optometry department, local supervisors, PQE examiners, optometrists, and dispensing opticians who have a special interest in certain aspects of optometry, to give tutorials or informal lectures. The emphasis should be on how best to apply theoretical knowledge in the practical environment of the examinations. The presenters' travel expenses and fees can be split among the group. Closer to the PQEs these meetings may be used to practice interview techniques, with the group analysing and criticizing individual performances. Local optometrists who are examiners should be invited to take part in these mock exam sessions.

During the year it is important to organize visits to factories or offices to examine the lighting systems and discuss aspects of safety eyewear with the safety officer. It is easier to describe a light or piece of safety eyewear in an examination if it has been previously seen and discussed. Organizations are more likely to arrange such visits for a group rather than on an individual basis. Local office blocks will also have a range of illumination, although it is doubtful whether anyone working there will have much knowledge of them. These places should be contacted as early as possible in the year, certainly before the December break. Local swimming pools, sports centres, train stations, and airports can be visited on a less formal basis, but it is unlikely that any of the workers will have knowledge of the illumination. However, the lighting can be described and discussed by the group.

4.2 COURSES

Most areas have a local optical society that organizes at least monthly lectures on topical clinical subjects. These are usually free to trainees and although not strictly aimed at the PQEs, provide up-to-date information as well as a good opportunity for you to meet fellow trainees and other optometrists working in your area.

The examinations are held in optometry departments. These vary each year and the CO will write to you with the venues that are being used in your examination year (see Chapter 2, p. 22). If you have a strong preference or your *alma mater* is one of the centres, then it is crucial that you reply to the CO and send your fees as soon as possible after you have received the application forms, preferably on the same day that the CO correspondence is received. There are obvious advantages in taking your examinations in your old department. These include familiarity with rooms, clinic set-up and equipment, familiar faces of lecturers (some of whom will also be examiners), technicians and sometimes patients, knowledge of parking, accommodation, and eating facilities.

Most of the optometry departments and the Institute of Optometry organize refresher courses directly aimed at the PQEs. These are usually held just before or just after the December break for the first set, and in April or May for the second set. Early application is advisable, as the courses do fill up quickly. However, it may be prudent to wait until CO notification of your examination centre. If this is not your old department, it may be beneficial to attend a refresher course at this centre. This will enable familiarization with the clinics and other amenities. If you are successful in registering for the examinations at your old optometry department, then it may also be wise to apply for a refresher course elsewhere, for it is very likely that your old lecturers will be heavily involved with the refresher course at your old department and some of the course notes may bear a striking resemblance to your undergraduate notes! A different approach and fresh notes from new lecturers may be useful.

It is probably a good idea to contact all of the organizations that run courses at the beginning of the year and ask to be put on their mailing lists (see Useful Addresses, p. 143). This will ensure that you do not miss out and that you are aware of costs and closing dates for applications.

5

Venues, accommodation, examination techniques, and communication

5.1 VENUES AND ACCOMMODATION

If you have been successful in registering at your old department then you will be familiar with the type and location of available accommodation. Those working for multiples will probably be resident in an all-expenses-paid-hotel. However, it is still important to know how far the hotel is from the department if it is in an area of the town that you are not familiar with. You may be able to stay with friends. Others will need to contact the university accommodation office for advice on accommodation. If this accommodation is unfamiliar, remember to ask about parking and the time it takes to reach the examination centre in the rush hour by car, public transport or foot.

If you are not attending your old department for the examinations you may still use this approach. The university accommodation office should be the first port of call, and it is again advisable to check on parking at the accommodation and the university, as well as travelling times to the department. Time is of the essence, so once the examination centre is known, accommodation should be arranged.

5.2 EXAM TECHNIQUE

It is better not to arrive too early, as this will result in more nerves. If there is plenty of time make sure you know your candidate number and the location of the room where your first examination will be held, then wait in another part of the building until a couple of minutes before you are due to be called. Then go and stand in the area where candidates are called from. There is only one thing to say about being late: don't be! A few deep breaths before going in may help. Dress smartly and don't go overboard on cologne or perfume. In fact it's best not to use any. White coats seem to have steadily gone out of vogue at the PQEs over the last few years and it is our opinion that it is not necessary to wear one. Long hair should be tied back.

When you enter the examination room, do not worry if an extra examiner is in attendance. He or she will probably be a roving examiner who will be assessing the performance of your examiners! The roving examiner will not take part in the examination process, but will sit silently and observe.

The examiners usually start with a couple of basic questions. Think before answering any question. Don't comment on your nervousness and don't use it as an excuse for lack of knowledge or poor performance. Always wait for the examiner to finish asking a question before you answer. Don't repeat the question out loud to yourself. Address your answer to the examiner who asked the question. Maintain eye contact, don't fidget or giggle, and never start with 'well, obviously'. Start with the basics and don't get too detailed too quickly. Remember the quicker you give the answer the more time there is for more questions. However, if you are deliberately slow the examiner will detect this and you will fail. Give detailed step-by-step answers and don't be obtuse.

Never say 'I don't know'. Give some information about something, but don't bring up areas that you don't know much about. Don't mention terms just because they sound good if you don't know what they mean or don't know any other details. Be honest and be sensible. Wait to be asked the next question and don't waffle, as this will annoy the examiner. Try to maintain a positive disposition towards the examiners, no matter how awkward or unfriendly they appear to be. Never argue. Always give the obvious answer and only talk about what you know about. The examiners want to know that you are safe to practice and not that you are the world's most knowledgeable optometrist. Don't just answer yes or no, give a discussion of the subject. Use only medical terminology and don't use lay terms. If you realize that you have made an error, the phrase 'That's wrong and this is what I meant to say . . .' is useful. The examiners are not there to help you. Recognize any flaw in your argument if pointed out to you and correct it. Be confident of your answer and stick with it if you are absolutely sure it is correct. If your answer is queried, you need to make an important decision. Have you said something wrong and the examiner is giving you a second chance? Is it a test of your confidence? Or is your answer not quite right and clarification is being sought? Be prepared to answer questions on relevant areas from other subjects, such as contact lens solutions in the drugs examination.

For those PQEs involving patients, even if they are undergraduate students, treat them as you would do in practice. Do not lose your temper or be rude in any way, even if the patient is being unco-operative. If confronted with an instrument you are unfamiliar with, say so and say what you would normally use. Know what you normally use well. Be safe in your answers and actions. It is a good idea to take a pen and paper into each examination. Even though the PQEs are mainly oral examinations, you may want to draw diagrams to help explain a point. Just to remind you, the CO regulations state that no books are allowed in the examination room!

After each PQE note as many questions as you can remember and the answers you gave. This will help later on if you have failed.

5.3 COMMUNICATION SKILLS

Success in your professional examinations is dependent upon a combination of good knowledge of the subject matter and the ability to apply this knowledge in a practical clinical situation. Unfortunately the time allowed for the candidate to both describe and demonstrate their knowledge is limited. This means the examiner has to make a judgement upon the candidate's performance based on sometimes as little as twenty minutes of contact. This inevitably means the decision will, at some level, be influenced by an overall perception of the candidate during this short period. As well as what is actually said by the candidate in answer to specific questioning, the way a candidate either answers or performs a certain task will always have some influence upon the outcome of 'live' (viva and practical) examinations.

Many candidates, when analysing reasons why they have not passed a particular part of their PQE, may often say 'I knew the answer but just could not explain it', or 'I answered that question but he/she still failed me on that point' or, worse still, 'He/she seemed to have it in for me'. The first two comments are obviously based upon a breakdown in communication, the last generally on a misinterpretation of behaviour (and never, in these days of well-trained and 'roved' examiners, a matter of personal animosity). Sadly there are many candidates each year who have been excellent as undergraduates, know the subject matter well, and yet fail because they just could not perform well on the day.

Furthermore, examiners may have to make a decision as to fitness to practise based upon limited information. Particularly in the case of a borderline candidate, this decision may be influenced by a judgement of clinical ability or confidence about the subject matter based upon the candidate's general performance. A shambling, erratic, nervous, and less than confident performance, even in the absence of any specific factual error or inaccuracy, may be sufficient to tip the balance against the candidate. To be fair, if the examiner has to judge a candidate as 'fit to practise' then a lack of confidence in carrying out a practical technique may be a sound criticism in many situations, particularly where patient management is concerned.

It is therefore very useful for all candidates to think carefully about all the factors other than a knowledge of the theoretical and practical syllabus (covered elsewhere in this book) that may influence the examiners' decision. Just as everyone reading this will be revising facts and technique, time spent on preparing one's 'performance' is time well spent. The bottom line is that, if you establish a certain rapport with the examiners, they will remember you in their post-assessment decision-making period in a more positive light.

Non-verbal behaviour

It is well established that, when communicating with another person in any situation, the amount of information transferred from one speaker to the other, and the proportion understood and retained by the listener, is significantly influenced by non-verbal behaviour. This refers to every action of the speaker other than that of actually speaking the words. Many research studies have established this pattern and it is particularly clear when a listener has been asked to make a subjective assessment of a speaker subsequent to an interview, when rating things such as confidence, predicted ability outside the interview room, professionalism, ability to cope in a crisis situation, and so on. One could add the perception of a candidate as 'fit to practise' to this list.

Before listing some of the non-verbal influences upon the examiner decision, it should be emphasized that nobody should ever be told exactly how to speak or present themselves. The world would be a very boring homogenous place indeed if such instructions were adhered to. However, if any particular mannerism or behaviour is influential, it is not only useful to understand this but some thought should be also given to how others may perceive us and, where this may be in a negative way, how this perception might be changed.

Appearance

You need to look professional. At the risk of sounding too conservative, it is likely that most examiners will expect you to look smart and well-presented. You might feel this to be a stereotype, but such an impression will convey that you will be presentable and acceptable to the public, who have to have a degree of confidence and trust in you, and that you also are likely to maintain certain standards of personal hygiene and self-respect that are generally considered essential for any clinical discipline. 'Professional' in this context is likely to mean business-like and most successful candidates, male or female, will wear smart suits.

On a different level, anything too distracting will influence, usually deleteriously, the examiner's recall of the examination when deciding afterwards upon the result. This may include particularly garish clothing or jewellery, unkempt or unusual hairstyles, or any provocative attire. Another point to remember is that occasionally, as will be restated later, certain physical attributes or mannerisms, particularly those beyond our control, need to be recognized and, where possible, minimized. A classic example is the flush of the upper chest and neck region many experience when nervous. A plunging neckline for such a person will only to serve to draw attention to this and unnecessarily distract, while at the same time enhancing the perception of nervousness that may detract from the overall performance.

Gestures and head-nods

Gestures, when speaking, are part of what makes us individual and certainly should not be suppressed. Indeed, there are many influences, both cultural and experiential, that influence every candidate's gestures and they often help to reinforce a message as much as to distract from it. However, it is always useful to be aware of what your body is doing when you are speaking. Most people seeing themselves speaking on video are surprised not only by how different their voice sounds, but also how animated their hand and head gestures often are. Identifying these gestures is useful as they can be controlled to some extent to, again, avoid too much of a distraction from what you are actually saying. This author is particularly prone to very stiff lips and a slight twitch when nervous; this is partly controlled by an occasional hand to the chin. Hand waving may be controlled if needs be by gently laying the hands, one over the other, on the knees (your own not the examiners!).

Head nodding is a well-established social signal that is used both to reinforce stated facts and, more importantly, to suggest when listening, that you are both attentive and understand what is being said. Examiners are occasionally unsettled when asking questions of a rigidly deadpan candidate, and the occasional head nod from the candidate helps to establish that all-important rapport.

Position and posture

The position relative to another person of a speaker gives much away in terms of authority of one person to another. This is unlikely to be easily influenced in an exam situation, as in most cases you will be seated opposite an examiner with a table in between. In practical situations, however, there may be more freedom, and standing too close to the examiner may be misconstrued as aggressive or confrontational. Furthermore, a very hunched or defensive posture is invariably interpreted as a sign of low confidence, whereas leaning forward across a table in a very extrovert manner may again be interpreted as aggressive. In general, an upright posture facing the examiner without leaning forward too obviously is a safe approach and can be easily rehearsed with your supervisor in your final mock exam sessions with them.

Eye contact

Eye contact is both a powerful influence upon interaction and perhaps the easiest to control once thought is given to it. In general, our social interactions throughout life establish an expected 'norm'. Generally, this is that when listening, you will usually maintain eye contact for the majority of the time (often as much as 90 per cent of the time spent listening), while much less of the time when actually speaking (typically 30 per cent or so). Bearing this in mind, if you maintain solid unbroken eye contact with someone when you are speaking to them, they will be distracted and generally feel uncomfortable enough not to take on board most of what you are saying. It may be interpreted as aggressive, or at the very least a sign of questionable emotional stability. Try staring hard at your supervisor next time you speak to them to confirm this! Once you are aware of this fact, you should be able to avoid inappropriate eye contact. If in doubt, imagine you are talking to a friend in a social situation and your eye contact is likely to reflect this less traumatic context.

When listening to a question, maintaining good eye contact throughout is useful. This will give the impression that you are attentive and listening, and add to the overall impression of confidence.

Primacy and recency

It is well established that the best-remembered parts of any interaction are those from the very beginning and the very end of the interaction. Bearing this in mind, remember that your initial welcoming greeting and parting farewell will have significant influence. If your opening gambit is 'I hate this subject' and your last statement is 'I really messed that up didn't I?' this will be on the examiners' minds when they attempt as objective a decision as possible about your performance.

Facial expression

There are two key components to controlling facial expression. First, do not let your facial expression (especially if accompanied by paralinguistic expressions such as sighs or tuts) betray your inner feelings. If you feel that a question is inappropriate or too easy or too hard, a frown or up-curled lip of disapproval will only break down any rapport, and occasionally create tension in the examination unnecessarily. Second, a very fixed expression, for example artificially happy or stiff through nerves, will again act as a distraction and, though it is not always easy, should be avoided. Try and adopt as close and natural an expression to your normal social self as possible.

Verbal behaviour (paralinguistics)

Paralinguistics is the psychologist's term for how something is said rather than what is said. It is especially important to be aware of it if you wish an examiner to feel you are confident about the knowledge you express.

Pitch and intonation

The 'music' of our speech is heavily influenced by regional accents, and again these are part of what make us individual and interesting. For example, a gradual increase in tone towards the end of a sentence is common to speakers from the north-east of England as well as to those from Australia. Putting this to one side, a gradual rise in tone accompanying a tailing off in volume often betrays a lack of confidence in an answer. Try saying 'I would refer this patient', first in a fairly constant tone and then with a rising tone and see which is the more convincing.

Speed and pacing

Many people will increase their speed of speech when nervous. This need not be a bad thing unless it leads to words being said before they have actually been thought through ('I shouldn't have mentioned that'). Very often, this is best controlled by allowing deliberate pauses between statements. As long as these do not extend into protracted periods of uncomfortable silence, they will have the benefit of allowing you to think about your next sentence, while at the same time allowing the examiner to digest what you have just said. Another obvious advantage is that the time of the actual exam will appear to go by much quicker! Practise sensible pauses in conversation with your supervisor.

The same theory might be applied to practical activities. A well-paced fluent approach to a technique, such as setting up a slit lamp, the examination of a low vision device or carrying out a tonometry reading, will convey a far more professional character. Remember, however, that it is a fine line between carefully taking your time and letting time drag!

Preparation and communication skills

The best thing you can do in the run-up to your exams is to practise. Get your supervisor or, perhaps even better, one of their colleagues with whom you are unfamiliar, to ask you some very general open questions. Good examples are 'Tell me all about diabetes and how it affects the eye', 'Discuss all the reasons why you might refer a cataract', 'Explain Snellen notation' and 'What is a phoria?' It is essential that the questions are open, i.e. have no single statement or fact as an answer. Though none of these should, in theory, present any problem, but if you have not rehearsed speaking out loud then, on the actual day, it may prove quite a task to get out all the information you wish to. It may require several follow-up questions from the examiner, leaving them with the perception that you are less sure of your subject.

It also allows you to develop the skill of explaining subjects in your own language. There is nothing worse from the examiners' point of view than a candidate explaining a concept (such as what a cotton wool spot actually is) by reciting verbatim from a handout or textbook. This is usually very obvious (occasionally a candidate even moving his/her eyes as if reading from the actual text!), such that the follow-up question is very often 'What does that all mean exactly?' This question is often left unanswered!

Having carried out this exercise, do not be afraid to ask the questioner not only whether your answers were acceptable but also if they felt you were confident in your response. Consider all the non-verbal and paralinguistic points raised here and see if any of them may have influenced the comments of your interrogator.

6

Re-takes

The CO will provide you with a brief report on why you failed a particular examination. Its usefulness will range from moderate to zero. Think back to the examination: you may be able to pinpoint the part(s) you failed on. Discuss failed PQEs at length with your supervisor. Go over those questions you had problems answering and make sure you can answer them if asked again in your re-take. It is unlikely that you will have the same examiner as on your first attempt, so it is possible that the same topics will be covered and that some questions may be very similar to those asked during your earlier attempt(s). Review the chapters in this book for the subjects you failed and look at the advice we give. Make sure you can answer all of the past examination questions for the sections you failed and revise the areas that the questions cover. Look at the examiners' comments on your failure report so that you know what to do and what not to do at the re-take!

September re-takes can be held at any of the optometry departments and some may hold re-take courses covering subjects that commonly lead to failure. The format is usually informal, small group tutorials.

Valuable extra experience can be gained on some topics, e.g. ocular disease and abnormality, anomalies of binocular vision, partial sight and its management, by attending primary care practices or hospital departments staffed by optometrists who specialize in these particular areas. See if you can arrange this in your locality. If not, be prepared to travel. Note these specialists may charge a fee for the time they spend with you.

The CO can provide counselling for candidates who fail a significant number of PQEs at the first attempt or who fail examinations at the second attempt (see Chapter 3, p. 29).

December re-takes (the third and final attempt for many trainees) are usually held at the Institute of Optometry, London. It is advisable to attend their re-take courses even if you have been before. If the outstanding PQEs are practical then do as much of that particular technique or techniques in your own practice as you can. Have several qualified optometrists observe and provide critical analyses of your work. If the outstanding PQEs are theory-orientated, study as much as possible and ask your supervisor and other qualified optometrists to viva you in a mock examination on a regular basis. It may be better to do less practice work and concentrate fully on the re-takes. It may also be useful to find another practice and another supervisor for this final attempt. If you fail any exams at the third attempt, you will have to wait 18 months before starting the whole cycle and re-take all ten PQEs. However, it is our experience that if you take our advice and prepare well, you are unlikely to end up in that position.

PART 2

A guide to the Professional Qualifying Examinations

Anomalies of binocular vision

Michelle Rundström and Martin Hodgson

7.1 WHAT DOES THE CO SAY?

The following information is taken from the CO pre-registration pack. The information in italics is our own and not provided by the CO. The syllabus is short and to the point: 'Normal and abnormal binocular vision, its development, assessment and management'.

The GOC provides a core curriculum/core competencies for BV (find it in your pre-registration pack supplied by the CO) and this will help you determine the standard you need to achieve in this subject.

The CO provides information under three headings: fitness to practise, nature of the examination and assessment.

7.1.1 Fitness to practise

'The qualified practitioner must be able to detect anomalies of binocular vision, to determine their aetiology as far as possible, to establish if there is a need for referral for a medical opinion, and to provide adequate management and advice to the patient.'

7.1.2 Nature of the examination

'The examination lasts for one hour and is in two parts. The first 30 minutes is spent with one examiner and comprises a practical investigation of the binocular vision of one or more patients. An oral with a second examiner lasts another 30 minutes and may range over the whole syllabus. The objective of both parts is to examine the candidate's understanding and clinical application of the basic principles of binocular vision.'

Either the practical or the oral could be first. In the practical examination, the candidate will be told the patient's refractive correction (including prisms if there are any) and will be expected to carry out an efficient and comprehensive assessment of the binocular status. The examiner will observe and may ask for clarification of specific points that arise. The investigation should demonstrate a logical selection of tests (conducting inappropriate tests will count against you), bearing in mind the history and symptoms, leading to a correct diagnosis and clear recommendations for management. An adequate selection of commonly used equipment will be available. (A sample of the record sheet to be used is on the CD-ROM provided by the CO.)

'A satisfactory practical must include the assessment of all appropriate aspects of history and symptoms as well as a range of suitable tests to determine the motor and sensory status of the patient.' *Work slowly and methodically through your examination and take care to make accurate observations. You can fail on one mistake. One of us (MH) failed this exam at the first attempt and the examiners' report simply stated, 'the candidate diagnosed an exophoria with great panache. Unfortunately the patient had a "tropia".*

'The oral examination. *This will range over the whole syllabus and may include some or all of the topics listed on the reverse of the examination record sheet.* 'You may be asked questions on any area of theory relevant to binocular vision, from visual development and anatomy to clinical techniques and management. There may be some overlap with other PQE topics, for example you may be asked about cycloplegics or about ocular diseases that may result in a binocular vision anomaly.'

7.1.3 Assessment

'In every case the examiners will look to see that the candidates have:

(i) Completed each procedure of patient examination in a smooth and logical order;

(ii) Demonstrated a command of techniques adequate to produce valid results;

(iii) Demonstrated a clear understanding of the results achieved;

(iv) Not failed to recognize any significant sign or symptom;

(v) Demonstrated in their final determination of each case a logical response to the particular history and symptoms, taking into account the legal and professional responsibilities of a practitioner;

(vi) Readily recognized and differentiated the concomitant and incomitant conditions;

(vii) A sound knowledge of the musculature and innervation of the extraocular muscles;

(viii) Indicated an understanding of the normal and abnormal development of acuity and binocular associations, in so far as these relate to the management of any anomalies;

(ix) A clear awareness of the criteria for referral.'

7.2 THE EXAMINATION FORMAT

The examination is split into two halves: a half-hour practical and a half-hour oral. Either can come first. One examiner will be present in each half of the exam and their combined decision will determine your result. It is possible to fail on mistakes made in only one half of the exam!

In the practical part you will be asked to examine one or more patients. Often this means two patients; we have never heard of any trainee being asked to see more than two. It is most likely that you will be asked to assess two patients; one long case and one short case. The long case will be the more involved of the two. You will be given the refractive error (including prism values) and you would be asked to examine the patient. An example of the type of anomaly you might encounter is a decompensated heterophoria or a fully accommodative esotropia. Following the history and symptoms, you should proceed to perform cover tests and an assessment of motility, followed by any other tests that are relevant to the case such as fixation disparity (aligning prism or sphere), determination of the sensory status and grading of the quality of binocularity, using for instance a stereoacuity test. At the end of the examination you will be expected to diagnose and describe the anomaly and state your management.

The short case will probably come second. As time is often running out you may simply be asked to perform one or two tests and comment on your observations. An example of this would be a patient with an extraocular muscle paresis. You may be asked to perform a cover test and assess ocular motility and be expected to observe an underaction, suggest which muscle might be affected and the associated muscle sequelae, and what the diagnosis might be. During the practical, the examiner will watch you closely but probably not interrupt. At the end he or she may ask you a few questions. Do not be afraid to ask the patient any relevant questions, as you would do in practice. If the patient's condition has previously been assessed they may even tell you what they have! But be careful, as patients are notoriously unreliable. Familiarize yourself with the record sheet used in the BV PQE. The CO will have sent a copy of this to you at the beginning of the pre-registration year.

In the oral part of the PQE a different examiner to the one who examined your practical will assess you. During the 30-minute assessment, questions will range from those requiring one word answers to those that require long explanations, such as explaining your management strategy for a given case. It has been known for candidates to be asked to interpret Hess plots. The same advice applies here as to the rest of the oral PQEs. Think carefully before you answer questions. Try to avoid referring to topics you know little about – some examiners may take your lead and decide to ask you more questions on a topic that you inadvertently mention. Only answer the question asked and do not waffle!

7.3 WHAT DO THE EXAMINERS SAY?

The following are comments provided by two PQE binocular vision examiners.

(a) What advice would you give to a candidate preparing for the exam?

A: Gain as much practical experience as possible. Extensive reading of current textbooks, papers and journals is important.

B: Be prepared to accept that you will probably not know the answer to all the questions asked; the examiner will either re-phrase the question or move onto another topic. In the practical, only do tests that are relevant and provide useful information.

(b) What areas of the subject require:

(i) Sound knowledge?

A: Methods of investigation. Classic anatomy of nerve pathways and muscles.

B: Actions of extraocular muscles and nerve pathways. Landmarks in visual development, e.g. visual acuity, fusion and stereopsis. Criteria for referral. Orthoptic therapy for convergence insufficiency, convergence excess and accommodative insufficiency. Classification of heterophoria and heterotropia. Management of strabismus and being able to differentiate between types that require surgical or conservative treatment or those that need a combination.

(ii) Reasonable knowledge?

A: Recent work and research on aetiology and nervous systems.

B: Syndromes, e.g. Brown's, Duane's. Tests for evaluation of BV, e.g. Bagolini lenses, stereopsis, Maddox rod, and Mallett unit.

(iii) Some knowledge?

A: Surgical techniques.

B: Surgical procedures. Examples of systemic and ocular diseases with associated BV problems. The risks associated with leukocoria.

(c) What do you look for in the successful candidate?

A: Attention to detail. Selecting clinically appropriate tests. Ability to recognize significance of findings and patients' responses.

B: Can the candidate think through the problems at hand and not give textbook statements? Not waffling when they do not know an answer and exposing their lack of knowledge. Having a clear understanding to take concise action in cases when patients need immediate referral.

(d) What brings marks down?

> A: Poor practical technique. Inability to interpret from what has been found in the practical.
>
> B: Candidates unsure of the answers they are giving. Performing tests that are inappropriate – this leads them to run out of time before making a diagnosis. Taking an excessively long time on the cover test and deciding what they want to see rather than what is actually there!

(e) What are the common causes of failure?

> A: Inability to recognize deviations and poor knowledge of consequences of binocular problems in infancy.
>
> B: Unable to correctly observe cover test movements. Incorrect diagnosis and treatment plan either in the oral or the practical. Unable to demonstrate clear knowledge of (i) extraocular muscle origins, courses, insertions, innervations, and actions (ii) landmarks in visual development (iii) orthoptic exercises and their application.

(f) What subject areas do candidates place too little importance upon?

> A: Anatomy and physiology, and sensory adaptations to deviations.
>
> B: Anatomy, vision therapy and vision development.

(g) Any other comments?

> A: The BV exam is NOT a monster. Most candidates have a very negative attitude to the subject and hence come in with a great amount of anxiety; this leads them to make uncharacteristic mistakes. Thinking of BV like other more 'enjoyable' subjects means that half the battle is won. Only answer questions that are asked (both in the practical and oral) and not those you would have like to have been asked.

7.4 HELP AND ADVICE

To follow on from one of examiner A's last comments, the binocular vision exam is often perceived as something of a monster! It need not be. With good theoretical and practical preparation during the pre-registration year, and some simple revision planning, you should enter the BV PQE with confidence.

In this section we will deal with the practical and oral sections of the BV PQE, then with how to gain experience in binocular vision assessment during the pre-registration year. It would be difficult here to cover in detail any plan of action for the practical. The next section is more of an ideas shower that gives our thoughts on what you might be thinking during the examination. During your revision consider the different types of BV anomaly that you might be faced with, and the best approach for each in terms of investigation and management.

7.4.1 The practical

Equipment to take to the exam

Click-on click-off pen torch, Romanes (guitar shaped) occluder, and detailed fixation targets, e.g. a reduced Snellen stick and a 6/60 letter printed onto an A4 sheet and attached to the back of a clipboard.

History and symptoms

Greet the patient and then explain that you will first ask some questions and then proceed to examine their eyes. This will instil confidence in the patient and help you to compose yourself. Have your questions planned. Be flexible and follow up any leads, e.g. if the patient reports diplopia, determine the mode of onset, duration, whether it is constant or intermittent, vertical, horizontal or oblique, with or without correction.

Note any associated head posture, ocular or non-ocular (if ocular, on straightening the head a deviation often becomes apparent). Note any obvious deviations, pseudo-strabismus (epicanthus, facial asymmetry, narrow or wide inter-pupillary distance), proptosis, ptosis or pupil anomalies. You can now proceed with your investigation, performing only those tests that are indicated by the patient's responses to your questions. Do not perform irrelevant tests, such as measuring stereoacuity on a patient with a constant large angle exotropia.

Investigation

Visual acuity

Measure vision and/or visual acuity (VA) using an appropriate method. You may need to perform a cover test with and without glasses, and therefore will need to know the vision and visual acuity. Measure binocular VA, which may be better than monocular VA in cases of latent nystagmus or worse if the patient is accommodating to overcome an exo-deviation.

Cover test

Choose suitable targets, distances and refractive correction if appropriate. Perform cover/uncover and alternate cover test and estimate the size of any deviation. Do not repeat the cover test *ad infinitum*; try to observe the movement with one or two tries. Do perform the cover test even if there is an obvious heterotropia.

Ocular motility

Observing corneal reflections test ductions if a mechanical restriction of movement is detected. Assess ocular motility and ask the patient to report any pain or double vision associated with eye movements. Use the alternate cover test in peripheral positions of gaze to determine the presence of any underacting muscles(s).

Other tests

Consider measuring motor fusional ranges, fixation disparity, stereopsis, Bagolini lenses, RAF convergence and accommodation, but only if you are familiar with using them. It is important to practise using a range of tests throughout the pre-registration year. Examiners can easily spot candidates who are not confident in their techniques.

Ask for any equipment you require. If you are not given the equipment you are used to, then say so but be prepared to answer questions on your own preference. For example, if you normally use a particular stereoacuity test, but are given an alternative then say why you prefer your usual test and know the specifications of it in detail. Sometimes the examiner may ask you not to do a particular test or may request that you carry out a specified test. Do not be concerned, you may just be running out of time and the examiner might want to see a specific test performed.

Conclusion

At the end of your investigation, give a diagnosis and description of the patient's condition, and outline how you would manage the case.

Management

Include prescribing advice, any necessary contact with the GP and recommend a re-test interval. Correct interpretation of your test results is important. It is unlikely that a patient sitting for your exam will require referral, as the condition is very likely to be longstanding and stable. Perhaps consider informing the GP, even if you are monitoring an anomaly yourself or it is long-standing and requires little or no action.

7.4.2 The oral

The list of past exam questions at the end of this chapter will give a good idea of the areas that you need to revise for this exam. The following list includes topics that are frequently examined:

- Development of vision and landmarks in visual development (VA, ocular movements, accommodation and stereoacuity among other things)
- Cranial nerve pathways (particularly third, fourth and sixth nerves)
- Brain stem anatomy, blood supply to head and neck

- Origins, insertions, functions and innervation of the extraocular muscles
- Sensory adaptation to strabismus
- Management of convergence and accommodative insufficiency
- Referral criteria
- Hess screen plots
- Brown's and Duane's syndromes, supranuclear and internuclear disorders
- Classification of heterophoria and heterotropia
- Orthoptic eye exercises
- Some knowledge of surgical treatment
- Detailed knowledge of commonly used clinical tests/equipment
- Know the advantages and disadvantages of your preferred tests and equipment
- 'Normal' values for heterophoria, fusional ranges and so on.

Also, at the risk of repetition:

1 Before answering questions, think carefully and logically, then give a concise reply that directly answers what is being asked. Avoid unnecessary statements and keep to the subject
2 Do not mention areas where your knowledge is weak
3 If you really do not know the answer to a rather specific and 'unimportant' question, it might be worth admitting it; the question will be rephrased or a new topic covered.

7.4.3 How and where to get experience

1 Incorporate as many practical techniques into your day-to-day eye examination routine as possible. This will improve your speed, accuracy and interpretation of results
2 Examine as many children as possible during the pre-registration year
3 Frequent visits to a local orthoptic department (or more than one department) are invaluable. You will see examples of simple routine tests carried out on patients with binocular vision problems. You will probably see more binocular vision anomaly cases in one day than in the whole pre-registration year in a high-street practice. You will also see orthoptists at work using techniques seldom used in optometric practice and gain an insight into the outcome of some of your referrals
4 Try to attend clinics with ophthalmologists who specialize in neuro-ophthalmology or binocular vision anomalies. You may have to travel to do this, but again in one day you could see a significant number of patients with conditions that you would otherwise gain little clinical experience of
5 Find a local optometrist who specializes in binocular vision anomalies and ask if you can attend one of their clinics
6 Attend relevant lectures at local optical meetings

7 If you are part of a student group (see Chapter 4), invite a speaker to talk to you about the optometrist's role in managing binocular vision anomalies.

7.5 PAST EXAM QUESTIONS

1 You see a ten-year-old child who, on initial examination appears to have a subjective refraction of right and left +1.00 DS. However, you saw right and left +3.00 DS on retinoscopy. What will you do next? What will you then prescribe?

2 Which VA test do you use in practice? What are its drawbacks?

3 You see an eight-year-old boy with VA of right 6/5 and left 6/12. He is fully corrected and wearing glasses constantly. Discuss your options for treatment.

4 What is internuclear ophthalmoplegia? Where is the lesion?

5 What is latent nystagmus?

6 What causes congenital nystagmus?

7 What is the level of vision at six months of age?

8 How would you measure vision in a child (a) <three years of age, (b) >four years of age?

9 Draw or explain the origin and insertion of the inferior oblique muscle. What action does it have?

10 Draw or explain the origin and insertion of the superior rectus muscle. What action does it have?

11 What is commonly associated with a superior rectus paresis? What is the reason for this?

12 Explain the concept of Panum's areas

13 In terms of angular subtense, how large are Panum's areas?

14 What is fixation disparity?

15 When fixing a near target, which is more accurate: accommodation or convergence? Which develops first, and at what ages do they develop?

16 An eight-year-old child has right and left +1.00 DS, a 20 prism dioptre (Δ) alternating exotropia at distance, a 15 Δ exophoria at near, accommodation of 18.00 DS at near with each eye, and near point of convergence 6 cm. How would you investigate and treat this case?

17 What is the level of stereopsis at six months of age?

18 Why is there an increased prevalence of esotropia in children at 3 to 5 years of age?

19 Why does strabismus sometimes occur after a bout of measles?

20 A 70-year-old patient reports sudden onset vertical diplopia. What questions would you ask during the history and symptoms and which are the muscles mostly likely to be affected?

21 A patient has a 30 Δ esotropia at distance and a 10 Δ esotropia at near. What are the possible causes of this anomaly? What is your course of action?

22 A 23-year-old patient presents with VA of right 6/5 and left 6/5, accommodation 13 DS each eye, no refractive error, no deviation at distance and 6 Δ esophoria at near. What symptoms may this person have? What would be your line of management? How would you discover whether the 6Δ esophoria is a problem to the patient?

23 Which nerves innervate the extraocular muscles?

24 Describe the pathway of the third cranial nerve.

25 Describe the pathway of the fourth cranial nerve.

26 Describe the pathway of the sixth cranial nerve.

27 What is the effect of a sixth cranial nerve palsy?

28 What would you see with a total third cranial nerve defect?

29 Describe the effects of a lesion at the fourth cranial nerve nucleus.

30 What are common causes of lesions of the third, fourth and sixth cranial nerves?

31 How would you manage (a) refractive amblyopia, (b) convergence excess?

32 Describe the development of the binocular vision system and give time periods.

33 What are the different components of the binocular vision system and how are they clinically assessed?

34 Your patient has a near decompensating esophoria. How would you assess this patient and what would be your management?

35 Your patient has a near decompensating hyperphoria. How would you assess this patient and what would be your management?

36 What are positive fusional reserves? What are normal base-in and base-out values at near?

37 What is meant by the term 'aligning prism'?

38 What are the signs of a partial third cranial nerve palsy?

39 How would you manage a child with a fully accommodative esotropia? Why is it important to prescribe the full refractive correction in these cases?

40 How do you know if a patient's hyperphoria is decompensating?

41 How would you investigate a librarian who complains of diplopia when placing books on a high shelf?

42 If a person presents with a ptosis and ipsilateral pupil dilation, what other test would you carry out?

43 Draw the muscle insertions and the centre of rotation of the eye

44 What problems would someone with a frontal bone blowout fracture have?

45 Why do most people have two eyes?

46 How would you modify your routine for a three-month-old child?

47 How would you modify your routine for a three-year-old child?

48 Why is the amplitude of accommodation usually greater with both eyes open than with each eye in turn?

49 What do you consider to be an abnormal near point of convergence?
50 What tests can be used to check for convergence insufficiency?
51 What is physiological diplopia? What is the difference between crossed and uncrossed?
52 Why is it considered more serious for a child to have an exotropia rather than an esotropia?
53 What are gaze palsies? What is their significance?
54 Describe Brown's syndrome and its features.
55 Describe Duane's retraction syndrome and its characteristics.
56 Describe this Hess plot.
57 What feature of this Hess plot indicates that the deviation is due to a restricted muscle and not a nerve palsy?
58 What is a common cause of a pain on eye movement?
59 A person has difficulty in looking up. What is the differential diagnosis?
60 What are the clinical features of microtopia and what would be your management of a six-year-old child with this diagnosis?

7.6 MORE INFO?

Eperjesi, F and Rundström, MM. *A Practical Guide to Binocular Vision Assessment*. Oxford: Butterworth-Heinemann, 2003.

Evans, BJW. *Pickwell's Binocular Vision Anomalies: Investigation and Treatment*, fourth edition. Oxford: Butterworth-Heinemann, 2002.

Evans, BJW and Doshi, S. *Binocular Vision: Evidence-based Assessment, Investigation and Management*. Oxford: Butterworth-Heinemann, 2001.

Ansons, A and Davis, H. *Diagnosis and Management of Ocular Motility Disorders*, fourth edition. Blackwell Science (UK), 2000.

8

Use of drugs in optometric practice

Martin Hodgson

8.1 WHAT DOES THE CO SAY?

The following information is taken from the CO pre-registration pack. The information in italics is my own and not provided by the CO. The syllabus is short and to the point: 'Properties, actions, selection, and use of drugs in optometric practice. Adverse reactions to topical and systemic medication.'

The GOC do not provide a specific core curriculum/core competencies for the use of drugs in optometric practice, but some information on standards can be found in the curriculum for Core Subject 3: Refractive Management (find it in your pre-registration pack supplied by the CO). This will help you determine the standard you need to achieve in this subject.

The CO provide information under three headings: fitness to practise, nature of the examination and assessment.

8.1.1 Fitness to practise

'When using drugs the qualified practitioner must be capable of:

(i)   Deciding which ophthalmic drugs are indicated
(ii) Administering them safely, responsibly, and with care and discrimination
(iii) Understanding the contra-indications, adverse effects and relevant safety measures.

In addition he or she must be able to recognize the ocular effects of local and systemic drugs where medication is reported or suspected.'

The words 'care and discrimination' are very important. Drugs must only be administered where necessary, and with care to choose the correct substance and concentration while being aware of potential side effects, adverse effects and safety measures. You should be seen as confident in your use of drugs, but take care to do so only when necessary and with a comprehensive knowledge of what you are doing.

8.1.2 Nature of the examination

The examination consists of a 20-minute oral with two examiners, one of whom will be an optometrist and the other usually a pharmacologist. Candidates may be asked questions relating to any part of the syllabus for this section. A selection of drugs, contact lens preparations and staining agents will be available for reference purposes.

8.1.3 Assessment

'In every case the examiners will look for:

(i)   An understanding of the pharmacological principles of drugs used in optometric practice;

(ii)   An ability to:
   (a) Recognize the indications for the use of a drug;
   (b) Select the most appropriate agent and appreciate the advantages and disadvantages of the selection;
   (c) Recognize significant findings and contra-indications (including interactions with systemic medication and clinical problems), and apply appropriate safety precautions and procedures;
   (d) Interpret the results of drug use.

(iii)   A knowledge of the preparations available for use in optometric practice and the principles underlying their formulation.

(iv)   An understanding of the signs and symptoms of the systemic effects from absorption after topical application or following accidental ingestion of ophthalmic drugs, and the action to be taken.

(v)   An awareness of the adverse and beneficial effects of local and systemic drugs on ocular integrity and visual performance, and of the appropriate action to be taken in relation to these effects.

(vi)   An understanding of the mechanism, signs, symptoms and management of allergic responses manifested in the eye from either topical drugs (including contact lens solutions), systemic drugs or environmental allergens.

(vii)   A knowledge of the use of drugs in the management of ocular emergencies.

(viii) A clear understanding of the legal constraints upon optometrists in relation to the use and supply of drugs.

This is an important area and the law governing the use of drugs by optometrists does not always provide a clear account that can be readily adapted to practical situations. Make sure you have a good idea of the types of practical situations in which you could, for instance, write a signed order to enable a patient to obtain therapeutic (prescription only) medicines from a pharmacist or in an emergency situation where you could supply therapeutic (prescription only) medicines directly to the patient.

(ix) A broad awareness of the drugs currently used in the treatment of ocular problems and diseases.'

8.2 THE EXAMINATION FORMAT

Two examiners will ask you questions for 20 minutes in total. There is no practical aspect to this examination and you will not have to carry out any procedures. The examiners will provide boxes of Minims, contact lens solutions, bottles of eye drops and other samples of ophthalmic drugs. Questions will be asked about these samples – you could be asked about the constituents of a contact lens solution or what the information printed on the packaging or bottle means. You will be asked general questions about your experience of using ophthalmic drugs in practice during your pre-registration year. Do not say that you have not used any!

Remember, commonly used substances such as fluorescein and saline are classed as drugs. You will be asked questions relating to the science behind drug use and questions relating to hypothetical clinical situations outlined by the examiners. You may be asked about the legal position of the optometrist in relation to the use and supply of drugs. You may be asked questions about ophthalmic drugs that cannot be used by the optometrist, for instance, drugs used in the treatment of glaucoma. You could also be asked about ocular side effects of systemic medication.

The examiners will generally be happy to re-phrase questions if you appear to have difficulty understanding what they are asking. Generally try to show that you have some experience using ophthalmic drugs in practice, that you are confident in doing so and that you have a sound knowledge of all aspects of the drugs you use. Do not try to impress the examiners by saying that you use drugs on virtually every patient. Despite the wealth of experience that this would have given you, it would also be seen as being rather reckless. You should only use drugs in practice if there is a clear indication for doing so, if it will lead to you gathering valuable data, if you cannot do this without using drugs, if there is very little risk to the patient, and if you know the possible adverse reactions and what to do if something does go wrong.

Don't worry if you think that you are getting a lot of questions wrong. In this examination, many candidates think they have done very badly and then find that they have passed! One examiner might be a pharmacist and ask questions that may seem theoretical or technical. It is likely that the optometrist examiner will not allow a wrong or 'don't know' answer to a question like this to fail a candidate.

8.3 WHAT DO THE EXAMINERS SAY?

The following are comments provided by three examiners:

(a) What advice would you give to a candidate preparing for the exam?

    A: Before the pre-registration year find out if your prospective supervisor stocks a range of optometric drugs and uses them regularly

    B: Carefully study the subject, especially the use of drugs in everyday practice. Know the drugs and solutions used, and carefully note patient medications during history and symptoms. Look up drugs you are unfamiliar with – this will gradually lead to a good understanding of the subject

    C: Read the syllabus – omit nothing

(b) What areas of the subject require

  (i) Sound knowledge?

    A: Working knowledge of basic optometric drugs. When to use them

    B: Drugs used in optometric practice. Pharmacology

    C: All parts!

  (ii) Reasonable knowledge?

    A: Pharmacology. Prophylactics

    B: Contact lens solutions. Drugs used in ocular therapy

  (iii) Some knowledge?

    A: Systemic drugs and possible ocular side effects

    B: Systemic side effects of ocular drugs

(c) What do you look for in the successful candidate?

    A: While a candidate is not expected by any means to have the breadth of knowledge that only experience will give, the person should have the ground data and be able to reason through the circumstances presented. Too often candidates have done so little basic ground work that they cannot be said to be safe to practise. If passed they receive a licence to practise for life!

    B: Sound knowledge and a demonstration of an interest in the subject, the ability to work out possible effects and side effects from basic pharmacology

    C: A safe approach and an understanding of the dangers inherent in all drug use

(d) What brings people's marks down?

    A: Candidates who are aware they are weak trying to slow down the examiners by dramatics and other delaying tactics. This leads to them being examined in more depth, as it causes suspicion that their knowledge may be flawed!

    B: Delaying tactics, waffle around the topic on which the question was asked or not answering a direct question

C: Not being prepared

(e) What are the common causes of failure?

A: Poor knowledge of the subject. Dangerous answers. For instance, one candidate stated that he would instil adrenaline for any patient with a red eye to make the eyes white, as this would satisfy the patient! This was said before he even mentioned checking the health of the eyes!

B: Lack of knowledge and reasoning ability, associated with a lack of interest. Not understanding the long-term implications of the examiners' decision

C: Not being safe

(f) What subject areas do candidates place too little importance upon?

A: Too often candidates are working in practices where the top priority is high income and too little importance is placed on teaching. The pre-registration year is supposed to be for adapting academic knowledge to good chair-side practice with the help of an experienced supervisor. Too often the candidate has been used as a cheap refractionist and given little training. A couple of days on a refresher course is not a substitute for proper training

B: Ocular effects of systemic medication. Emergency treatment. Contact lens solutions used in practice. In many cases candidates do not even know what percentage of saline is in cans or the percentage hydrogen peroxide in disinfecting solutions that are given to patients or the effects if these are accidentally instilled into the eye

(g) Any other comments?

A: Too often candidates seem to have done little work during their pre-registration year. Hands-on experience followed by discussions with your supervisor are extremely valuable. Often a candidate has not put a drop of anything into an eye, let alone seen what happens, has been encouraged not to refer too many people, has never put a contact lens in an eye, and has never seen a patient through from initial fitting to final aftercare. If they haven't done it, how can they have gained the knowledge and experience for us to pass them as safe to practice?

This may seem exaggerated but our experience indicates it isn't! It does show that the examiners sometimes have grave doubts about candidates having gained sufficient experience. Try to put across in the examination how much experience you have gained during your training year

B: Examiners are not looking for 100 per cent correct answers. The candidates should be prepared to say 'I don't know', if unable to answer or ask for the question to be clarified. Obviously if this happens too frequently it will be interpreted as a lack of knowledge of the basic subject.

8.4 HELP AND ADVICE

To meet the main requirements of the examiners, you must do the following:

1 Show that you have had experience of using drugs in practice.
2 Demonstrate a confident but discriminating and safe approach to the use of optometric drugs.
3 Have a sound knowledge of all the drugs you use and contact lens solutions that you recommend to patients.
4 Have reasonable knowledge of the ophthalmic preparations and contact lens solutions available, basic pharmacology and ocular reactions to systemic drug use.

From the above list you will be able to see that in order to prepare for this examination, you must first gain as much experience as possible during your training year of using optometric drugs. Ask your supervisor to allow you to examine any children who might require cycloplegic refraction, or diabetics who may require dilation. Think carefully about which contact lens solutions you should recommend; choose two or three types for soft lenses and two or three for gas-permeable lenses. Make sure you have clear reasons for why you have chosen them as your solutions of choice and know everything about them. For example, do you know the constituents of each? Where necessary ask the manufacturers for technical information.

The second requirement for this examination is a sound knowledge of the subject. It will be extremely useful for you to look at the list of past examination questions at the end of this chapter. The questions at the end of this chapter will give you a good idea of the areas you should revise before hand. Know the theory and think about it in relation to clinical practise. Plan in your mind what you would do in a variety of clinical situations. For example, what would you do if you needed to dilate but the patient has a very narrow anterior chamber angle? Would you know what to do if a patient develops adverse reactions to any of the drugs you use? Know that drug action times vary, but know roughly how long the drugs you use take to achieve maximum effect and recovery times. Know contra-indications, precautions to be taken, advice to be given to the patient and possible side effects. Mention that occluding the caniculli after drop instillation can reduce the chances of a systemic adverse reaction. Know if any systemic drugs could react with the topical ones you use. Find out from your local eye casualty department if they would recommend that you use drugs in emergencies before referral. Know systemic drugs that cause ocular side effects, the conditions for which they are prescribed and the effects that they cause. Know the law relating to drug use by optometrists.

There is to be a change in this examination. Beginning with the examinations sat in 2005, Use of Drugs will be merging with one (as yet undecided) of the other examinations.

8.5 PAST EXAM QUESTIONS

1 What drugs have you used in practice?
2 What cycloplegic would you use on a two-year-old child?
3 What precautions must be taken with the use of atropine?
4 Why does fluorescein fluoresce?
5 What drug groups may result in ocular adverse reactions? Give examples of drugs in these groups?
6 What would you look out for if a patient were taking steroids?
7 Why are betablockers prescribed for glaucoma? How do they work?
8 What topical anaesthetic would you choose for corneal anaesthesia prior to conducting contact tonometry? Why?
9 How does a mydriatic such as tropicamide work?
10 Why is tropicamide available in two doses?
11 What does 'Ph Eur' stand for on a Minims box?
12 What ocular adverse reactions may occur with systemic drug x?
13 Is the contraceptive pill a steroid?
14 What ocular adverse reactions may occur with steroids?
15 What precautions would you take before instilling a mydriatic?
16 What methods are available for checking whether the anterior chamber angle is open or closed?
17 Which anti-infectives available to optometrists may not be sold or supplied to a patient under any circumstances?
18 Which anti-infectives are antibiotics and what are the problems associated with the use of antibiotics?
19 What is a signed order?
20 What adverse reactions may occur with chloramphenicol?
21 What are the different components of contact lens solutions?
22 What are the components of Minims?
23 What are the components of dropper bottles?
24 Why do eye-drops sting?
25 How are Minims sterilized?
26 Which eye-drops sting?
27 What volume of drugs does a Minim hold?
28 What drugs could you instil if you precipitate an attack of closed angle glaucoma (CAG)?
29 What would you do if you precipitated an attack of CAG?
30 Describe the signs and symptoms of open angle glaucoma (OAG) and CAG?
31 What is the differential diagnosis of red eye in CAG and iritis?
32 Why is cyclopentolate used in the treatment of iritis?
33 What protein-removing solutions do you use?
34 Are there any advantages of using one type of contact lens solution instead of another?

35 What non-preserved systems do you know of and how do they work?
36 Do hydrogen peroxide contact lens solutions contain a preservative?
37 Is fluorescein a drug? How does it work?
38 What is Rose Bengal? When is it contra-indicated?
39 Are there any side effects associated with chloramphenicol?
40 Why is fluorescein usually in single dose disposable form?
41 How much fluorescein is absorbed in a single fluoret?
42 Define the following terms: (a) clean, (b) disinfect, (c) sterilize, (d) sanitize. Give examples of each method
43 Would the above methods be effective against: (a) virus, (b) fungus, (c) micro-organisms, (d) bacteria?
44 What drugs could be used prophylactically following corneal trauma? Can these be obtained from a pharmacist without a prescription?
45 Can an optometrist prescribe ocular therapeutics?
46 What is folic acid and where does it come from? What is the chemical process?
47 How are most modern all-in-one contact lens solutions preserved?
48 What is the difference between bacteriostatic and bactericidal?
49 What is the mode of action of an antibiotic?
50 When can chloramphenicol be used?
51 What miotics are available to optometrists?
52 When would you use a mydriatic? When would the use of a mydriatic be contraindicated?
53 Describe a Minims box?
54 What is meant by 'USP, BP, w/v, and DOM'?
55 How does a drug get from topical instillation to the site of action?
56 How much arrives at the site of action by each technique?
57 What is meant by drug specificity, ionic, equilibrium, selective toxicity?
58 What are the signs and symptoms of atropine poisoning? What is the cause? What is the cure?
59 Is atropine still used?
60 What would happen if a patient took an overdose of physostigmine?

8.6 MORE INFO?

Pearson, R and Hopkins, G. *O'Connor Davies' Ophthalmic Drugs: Diagnostic and Therapeutic Uses*, fourth edition. Oxford: Butterworth-Heinemann, 1998

Doughty, M. *Ocular Pharmacology and Therapeutics*. Oxford: Butterworth-Heinemann, 2000.

College of Optometrists. Optometrist's Formulary, No. 2, CO, 1994.
    (On the CD-ROM in pre-registration pack supplied by CO.)

Investigative techniques

Ian Moss

9.1 WHAT DOES THE CO SAY?

The following information is taken from the CO pre-registration pack. The syllabus is very short and to the point: 'Techniques employed during optometric investigation.'

The GOC do not provide a specific core curriculum/core competencies for investigative techniques but some information on standards can be found in the curriculum for Core Subject 5: Ocular Examination and Technique (find it in your pre-registration pack supplied by the CO). This will help you determine the standard you need to achieve in this subject.

The CO provide information under three headings: fitness to practise, nature of the examination and assessment.

9.1.1 Fitness to practise

'The qualified practitioner is expected to be able to determine from the patient's history, signs and symptoms and other relevant findings, the need of those cases for **tonometric investigation, visual fields investigation, and slit lamp examination**. The significance of colour vision defects, tests and methods for their detection must be understood and the relevance of contrast sensitivity tests in optometric investigation appreciated. A practitioner may reasonably be expected to have an understanding of those techniques which may be carried out on a patient referred for further investigation, including electrodiagnosis, ultrasonography, external and internal eye photography.'

9.1.2 Nature of the examination

'The examination comprises both oral and practical elements lasting one hour, with two examiners. The oral, which may occupy approximately 30 minutes at the discretion of the examiners, will cover the more theoretical aspects of the syllabus. Practical elements will occupy the remaining time, with emphasis on familiarity with the three primary techniques employed, including the adoption of safe procedures and appropriate follow-up. Patients are provided, and a selection of instruments and equipment will be available.'

9.1.3 Assessment

'In every case the examiners will look to see that candidates have demonstrated a safe, clinical awareness of the investigative techniques indicated and/or employed in optometric practice, and have:

(i) An awareness of the place of and indications for the investigation employed.

(ii) A knowledge of the relevant anatomy and physiology, and their significance with respect to observations.

(iii) A sufficient practical command of techniques adequate to produce valid results and a proper understanding of the findings, which may include the interpretation of specimen visual field defects and other records of clinical investigations.

(iv) Adequate control of the examination of a patient.

(v) A logical response to the results, taking into account the practitioner's legal and professional responsibilities, with particular reference to referral for medical and/or ophthalmological investigation.

(vi) An awareness of the advantages of a wide range of instruments and techniques, acquaintance with the range of methods normally available and, where relevant, supplementary techniques and equipment used.'

9.2 THE EXAMINATION FORMAT

As described in the previous section the examination is divided roughly into two parts. The principles of all aspects of tonometry should be known and its role in the detection and management of glaucoma. You will be asked particularly about the instrument you have used in practice. You must therefore be aware of the principle of how it works, and in the case of non-contact tonometry, what the additional buttons are used for.

Particular attention should be drawn to patterns of visual field loss and the visual pathway. The optic chiasm and associated structures are commonly referred to and an anatomical drawing is often asked for. Other subject areas such as colour vision, contrast sensitivity, ultrasound, photography, and electrodiagnostic testing are discussed, usually towards the end of the section. For the practical parts, do not carry out procedures in the examination that you have never practised elsewhere. Inexperience is obvious to the examiner, especially if you have stated that this is a technique you perform on every patient.

Questions are usually graded according to whether they are pass or fail questions, or if the examiner has decided you are worthy of a pass, then which grade you will be awarded. If you think you are being asked difficult or obscure questions you have probably done well.

Tonometry

You will be asked to perform tonometry on a patient. This constitutes usually one eye only, but proceed to record both eyes unless otherwise requested by the examiner. Remember to check that your instrument is correctly calibrated, and if you use the American Optical Non-contact Tonometer, that it is correctly focused for you and the patient. Talk to the patient, as you would do in practice. You are likely to be asked additional questions during your measurement procedure. For contact tonometry remember hygiene, drugs and implications.

Slit lamp

You will be asked to demonstrate several types of illumination. Before asking the patient to the chin-rest remember to check the set-up of the slit lamp; it may have been left untouched from the previous candidate, e.g. dissociated, wrong filter, and check the magnification. Additional techniques for the slit lamp may then be discussed, e.g. gonioscopy and anterior chamber examination, fundus examination, pachymetry, aesthesiometry, and other such topics.

Visual fields

You may be asked to establish central threshold on a semi-automated instrument. You may not be given the choice of which instrument to use, so be familiar with as many different types as you can. You might, however, be given the choice of using any one of several instruments in the examination room.

9.3 WHAT DO THE EXAMINERS SAY?

You must have an understanding of all of the equipment available in your practice, i.e. slit lamp, tonometer, visual field analyser, and colour vision tests. If you say you have used a certain instrument you must be aware of how it works, what all the buttons are used for, and what are its limitations and advantages over other similar instruments. The role of the optometrist in the detection and follow-up of glaucoma is particularly important in this examination.

Subject areas requiring particular attention are: ophthalmic equipment, visual pathways and interpretation of field plots' sensitivity, and specificity of diagnostic techniques for glaucoma management, e.g. the limitations of using only tonometry as a diagnostic test without optic disc assessment or visual field investigation, referral criteria for glaucoma.

What the examiners look for:

1 Smooth, logical and competent instrument skills.
2 The ability to make safe decisions and with justification when a hypothetical clinical situation is described, e.g. when to refer?
3 The ability to demonstrate that all techniques are as routine as possible.

Difficulty with any of the above is a common cause of failure. In particular, the inability to make correct clinical decisions, e.g. tonometry is not just about recording intraocular pressure on a record card. Know how to interpret the information once you have recorded it.

9.4 HELP AND ADVICE

This is one of the most important examinations, allowing you to be logical and realistic in your ability to make clinical decisions. Compared to other practical examinations, this is one you can most prepare for beforehand. A common cause of failure is poor use of the equipment that has supposedly been used frequently through the training period. Use a slit lamp, tonometer and visual field analyser as much as possible. Ask your supervisor to critically review your routine on a number of patients. Attend at least one refresher course, preferably at your examination centre. Ask someone if you are not sure of anything. Do not wait until the examination to be caught out!

The guidelines as to when to refer a patient are more of a grey area. There is no defined set of rules, since these vary from one referral centre to another. You must be sure in your own mind as to when and when not to refer, particularly for glaucoma and ocular hypertension. Talk with the ophthalmologists in your location and find out when they would like you to refer glaucoma suspects.

Patient management is very important in this PQE. The examiner wants to see and know what you intend to do with the patient. Treat the patient as you would in practice.

Some of the points described above may seem trivial, but if forgotten in the time-pressured examination situation could result in failure. The best way to prevent this is to be prepared by working to the examination format beforehand. The next section will give you an idea of potential questions or tasks. There are a number of questions to which there isn't a single correct answer. A course of action is determined by clinical competence and judgement. Whatever your final decision you must know what you are doing, why you are doing it and the implications for your patient.

9.5 PAST EXAM QUESTIONS

Tonometry

1 What tonometer do you use and why?
2 What is the Imbert–Fick law?
3 How does the Keeler Pulsair work?
4 How does the American Optical Non-Contact Tonometer (AONCT) work?
5 What do you do before using the AONCT?
6 How do AONCT values compare to values recorded with contact tonometers?
7 What physiological factors influence intra-ocular pressure (IOP)?
8 Demonstrate how you would check the calibration of this AONCT.
9 Demonstrate how you would check the calibration of the Keeler Pulsair.
10 What do you do after IOP measurement?
11 When would you measure IOP?
12 Describe briefly the mechanism for aqueous production and drainage.
13 Which drugs can affect IOP?
14 How would you manage a patient whose IOP was 26 mm Hg in each eye?

Slit lamp

15 When would you use a slit lamp in practice?
16 What attachments are available for a slit lamp?
17 What are the different illumination techniques and what would you use them for?
18 Demonstrate a given viewing technique.
19 Demonstrate Van Herrick's technique.
20 What is the principle of gonioscopy?
21 Describe the anatomy of the anterior chamber?
22 How could the fundus be examined with the slit lamp?
23 How is the slit lamp used in contact lens fitting?
24 Describe in brief your slit lamp routine for a contact lens aftercare.
25 What filters are available on your slit lamp?
26 What auxiliary lenses are available for use with the slit lamp?
27 What parts of the retina can be examined using auxiliary lenses?

Visual field analysis

28 What visual field analyser do you use in practice and what are its advantages and disadvantages?
29 When would you examine the visual field?
30 What is the extent of the normal binocular visual field?

31 What are the dimensions and location of the 'blind spot'?
32 Describe the differences between static and kinetic visual field testing?
33 What might cause:
    (a) Bitemporal hemianopia?
    (b) Binasal hemianopia?
    (c) Quadrantic field defect?
    (d) Ring scotoma?
    (e) Nasal step?
    (f) Arcuate scotoma?
34 What are the main blood vessels surrounding the optic chiasm?
35 What is the extent of the monocular visual field?
36 What is the difference between a positive and a negative field defect?
37 Draw and comment on a selection of field plots.
38 What is the difference between threshold and suprathreshold visual field analysis?
39 What are the common causes of artefacts that can affect a visual field plot?
40 What is the best method of screening the macular?
41 What is macular sparing?
42 What toxins cause visual field loss and what part of the field is classically affected?
43 What is meant by the term 'disproportion'?
44 What are the visual field requirements for driving?
45 How does visual field testing for driving differ from conventional testing?
46 Do you know the name of a visual field test specially designed for assessing drivers?
47 Describe in brief a non-automated method for assessing visual fields.

Other topics

48 What is the incidence of colour vision deficiency in males and females?
49 When would you test colour vision in practice?
50 What are the advantages and disadvantages of each type of colour vision test?
51 What are the effects of tungsten lighting on the colour vision testing? What lighting should be used?
52 What ocular conditions result in acquired colour vision defects?
53 Describe the D–15 test.
54 Does contrast sensitivity have a role to play in optometric practice?
55 What is the difference between a-scan and b-scan ultrasonography? What are their clinical applications?
56 Draw the Circle of Willis.
57 Draw the pathway of the nerves involved in pupil reflexes?
58 Given particular pupil defects, where could the causative lesion be?

59 What applications do electrophysiological techniques have in optometry and ophthalmology?
60 What are your referral criteria for suspected glaucoma?

9.6 MORE INFO?

Elliott, D. *Clinical Procedures in Primary Eye Care*, second edition. Oxford: Butterworth-Heinemann, 2003.
Henson, D. *Optometric Instrumentation*. Oxford: Butterworth-Heinemann, 1994.

Partial sight and its management

Frank Eperjesi

10.1 WHAT DOES THE CO SAY?

The following information is taken from the CO pre-registration pack. The information in italics is my own and not provided by the CO. The syllabus is short and to the point: 'Legal and welfare considerations concerned with visual standards. Epidemiology and management of impaired vision.'

The GOC do not provide a specific core curriculum/core competencies for partial sight and its management but some information on standards can be found in the curriculum for Core Subject 3: Refractive Management (find it in your pre-registration pack supplied by the CO). This will help you determine the standard you need to achieve in this subject.

The CO provide information under three headings: fitness to practise, nature of the examination and assessment.

Fitness to practise

'The qualified practitioner must be able to assist partially sighted patients providing advice on suitable visual aids and their use, utilization of residual vision, the benefits of available welfare services and the need for rehabilitation or retraining.' *During the examination the examiner will decide if the candidate is safe to practise with low vision patients.*

Nature of the exam

One examiner undertakes the 20-minute oral examination. No patients are provided but relevant equipment may be available for discussion. *There is always a selection of low vision devices on hand, some of which the candidate is asked to comment on. (See next section on examination format.)*

Assessment

The candidate must show:

(i)   An understanding of the underlying causes of visual impairment and the application of specialist knowledge in providing assistance. *The main ophthalmological causes of low vision and their signs and symptoms must be known well.*

(ii) An ability to recognize those patients who will benefit from assessment or advice supplementary to the basic routine, and the optometrist's responsibilities to such patients.

(iii) An awareness of the means by which such assessment or advice may be obtained nationally and locally. *Know where to obtain social care information and where to direct the patient.*

(iv) A familiarity with various visual aids available and the optical properties of their design. *This could involve ray diagrams!*

(v)   An understanding of the advantages and disadvantages of various types of low vision aid, their particular application and suitability for hypothetical patients.

(vi) A knowledge of legal definitions and regulations pertinent to the visually handicapped. *This information is in the Association of Optometrists handbook.*

10.2 THE EXAMINATION FORMAT

As mentioned above there is only one examiner for this PQE and no patients. There will be a desk between the candidate and the examiner, on which there may be a selection of low vision devices, near acuity charts, contrast sensitivity charts and Amsler grids. Equally these may be on a table adjacent to the interview desk or even behind the examiner, out of your view. During the 20 minutes of the exam the examiner will ask a range of questions, possibly in the form of case studies or questions covering a certain topic, such as diseases that cause low vision. All areas of low vision will be covered. Any low vision device may be presented for comment. Ray diagrams may have to be drawn for which paper and a pencil will be provided.

10.3 WHAT DO THE EXAMINERS SAY?

The following are comments provided by three examiners.

(a) What advice would you give to a candidate preparing for the exam?

   A: Read around the subject. Know how to access local rehabilitation services. Never start by saying you have not seen any low vision patients. All candidates will have seen some low vision patients even if they just required a high add and advice on appropriate lighting.

B: Read the syllabus, omit nothing and try to prepare for obvious questions.

C: Work very hard; those who pass have greater knowledge. Think about presentation and communication skills. Treat the PQE like an interview. Practise the exam situation.

(b) What areas of the subject require
   (i) Sound knowledge?
       A: Assessment of patient, vision; refraction and magnification. Referral protocols, procedure, timing, and local variables. How to evaluate a low vision device never seen before. Know exactly how hand and stand magnifiers work.

       B: All parts; a candidate could be failed on any part. A detailed knowledge is required for low vision aids, optics, advice, referral, problems caused by eye disease, and the registration process.

       C: I would not try and lead candidates along any particular path of knowledge in this or any other subject. Those who pass demonstrate good all-round knowledge. In general, stick to basics.

   (ii) Reasonable knowledge?
        A: Other low vision optics, epidemiology and statistics.
        B: Social and voluntary provision.

   (iii) Some knowledge?
        A: Other personnel involved in low vision. Their existence and roles but not necessarily what they do. Electronic and non-optical devices.

(c) What do you look for in the successful candidate?
       A: I imagine they are being let loose on my 85-year-old grandmother, who lives alone and wants to remain independent. If I think she would leave the consultation with better advice and knowing where next to go, then I would pass the candidate. If I felt that she would leave with the same or more difficulties, then they would fail.

       B: A good all-round approach. The candidate should be able to tackle a problem and think on his or her feet.

       C: Good communication skills, all-round knowledge. A sense that they would be able to deal with the real life situation.

(d) What brings people's marks down?
       A: Saying they have never seen a low vision patient. They have dug a deep hole and it's uphill from there on. The candidate has

a responsibility to have seen at least some, even if only for hand magnifiers or lighting advice.

B: Not being prepared.

C: Lack of knowledge or inability to put over their knowledge.

(e) What are the common causes of failure?

A: An apparent lack of thought and dismissive lack of interest. Inability to assess an unfamiliar optical device.

B: Not being prepared.

(f) What subject areas do candidates place too little importance upon?

A: The simple practical and realistic aspects of assessment, devices and referral.

B: Most of them!

C: Pre-preparation by rehearsing the PQE situation with their supervisor or friend. They should become used to being asked and answering questions.

(g) Any other comments?

A: If I ask what is the benefit of registration and another candidate replies with 'you get £1.25 off a TV licence', I will scream. The broad gains in rehabilitation terms and provision for special needs are much more important. Too many candidates feel that once they have referred their job is over. They should carefully differentiate between referral for rehabilitation and referral for pathology, and be prepared to advise on the former as their own responsibility, even if it means referral to another optometrist or a social worker. The referral route via GP to ophthalmologist is a legal entity but also in this case can be a cop-out.

10.4 HELP AND ADVICE

The following are important points or areas that need to be covered in preparation for the Partial Sight and Its Management PQE.

Optical

Expect to be shown a selection of low vision devices at some stage in this examination. The more devices you have seen in your pre-registration year, the greater the chance that you will recognize these and be able to comment correctly on them. A working knowledge of the Keeler low vision set and other commonly available magnifiers is paramount. The candidate should be able to reproduce ray diagrams of Galilean and astronomical telescopes, and hand and stand magnifiers. It is important to know what type of spectacle prescription, i.e. distance or near, to use with each particular type of magnifier. Most stand magnifiers have divergent emergent vergence so they need to be used in conjunction with a reading add for a presbyopic patient. The accommodative amplitude would need to be taken into account for a pre-presbyopic patient. Many hand magnifiers have one curved and one flat side. The flat side should be towards the face if the working distance is less than the focal length, and away from the face if the working distance is greater than the focal length. In all cases the magnifier should be held as close as possible to the eye to produce a large field of view.

The candidate should be familiar with the use of the Bailey–Lovie distance and near acuity charts and why they are considered to be better than the Snellen chart, especially in the field of low vision. Some familiarity with the Pelli–Robson contrast sensitivity chart is also required.

Knowledge of the use of non-optical devices such as CCTVs, contrast enhancement, illumination, and the Prentice typoscope is required.

Pathology

You should be familiar with the incidence, prevalence, and visual symptoms caused by common types of acquired and congenital ocular pathology, e.g. age-related macular disease, cataract, glaucoma, diabetes, and albinism. The major causes of registration in the young and old are required. Re-referral criteria for those patients previously discharged from the HES are necessary.

Social care

Criteria for full and partial registration, and the benefits both nationally and in your locality should be known well. Remember that registration is not a prerequisite for applying for help from social services. Talking books can be obtained for a fee if the person is not registered blind or partially sighted, but the fee is waived for those who are registered. It's up to you to find out where your local social worker for the visually impaired is based and ask to go on a home visit. Find out what other types of rehabilitation facilities are available in your area.

Miscellaneous

You may be presented with some case histories and asked to comment on the management for that particular person. Those working in general practice may not gain much experience of working with low vision patients, so it is advisable to visit a voluntary low vision centre or a hospital low vision clinic several times during the year. This will expose you to the low vision patient, their problems and the equipment.

There is to be a change in this examination. Beginning with the examinations sat in 2005, Partial Sight and its Management will be merging with one (as yet undecided) of the other examinations.

10.5 PAST EXAM QUESTIONS

1 How would you carry out refraction on someone with low vision, e.g. best visual acuity 6/60?
2 What are the advantages and limitations of a telescopic low vision aid (LVA)?
3 What is eccentric viewing?
4 What advice would you give to an older person living on their own who has age-related macular degeneration (AMD)?
5 What help is there in your area for partially sighted and blind people from social services and other groups?
6 What are the classifications of partial sight?
7 If a patient can read N24 with a +4.00 DS add in the trial frame, what power of magnifier do they need to read N6?
8 What visual problems is a person with retinitis pigmentosa (RP) likely to have?
9 What are the legal definitions of blindness and partial sight?
10 How would you define a LVA?
11 What is the main cause of blindness in the over 65-year-olds?
12 What level of visual acuity would you expect with AMD?
13 What size of area on a page of print would be lost with AMD?
14 How is the technique of eccentric viewing taught?
15 What are the visual standards to be registered partially sighted?
16 What financial benefits are available on partial sight registration?
17 What types of LVA have you dispensed in practice?
18 What advice on partial sight have you given?
19 What near VA would you expect with 6/36 in each eye?
20 What facilities are available for blind people in your area?
21 What is the blind registration form called and what sections does it have?
22 Who receives each copy?
23 What sort of help does social services provide?
24 Define blindness and partial sight?
25 What benefits are available?
26 What routine would you follow for this type of patient?
27 What is the difference between an astronomical and a Galilean telescope?
28 How would you help a person with albinism at work? What symptoms do they complain of?
29 What would you do to help a patient with problems of mobility?
30 How would you advise low vision patients' relatives to write letters to them?
31 How are these LVAs used? (Shown a selection of LVAs)
32 What is the difference between a ×3 spectacle magnifier and a hyperocular?

33 Which gives the highest magnification, a Galilean or an astronomical telescope?

34 What lenses are in these telescopes? (Shown a selection of telescopes)

35 Why do some Galilean telescopes have more than two lenses?

36 How can a standard Galilean telescope be changed for use at near?

37 Do you decrease or increase the distance between the lenses of a Galilean telescope to decrease the working distance?

38 With a stand magnifier, do you advise the patient to keep their reading glasses on or off?

39 What sort of refractive error do people with albinism usually have?

40 What is the dioptric power of these two magnifiers? (Shown two magnifiers with the magnification written on each)

41 Is near acuity or mobility taken into account during the registration process?

42 Who is the only professional who can register a person with low vision?

43 What magnifier do you recommend most and why?

44 How is the magnification of a Galilean telescope determined?

45 Are RP sufferers photophobic?

46 What is a CCTV assessment? Who can recommend patients for them? Which professionals are involved?

47 Do RP sufferers prefer white on black or black on white text when using a CCTV?

48 How would you help a person with albinism see a VDU screen?

49 Demonstrate how this CCTV works. (Shown a CCTV)

50 An 80-year-old patient with AMD, small pupils, clear media, no glasses, R6/60 L3/60 and N24 when binocular at near, wants to read the newspaper. How do you go about your routine?

51 What sort of acuity charts do you use and at what distance? Are there any special charts for near and distance acuity for the low vision patient?

52 What distance and power of lens is required for use with the Bailey–Lovie near word card?

53 A patient has N24, how would you calculate the power of magnifier that would enable the patient to read N6? What LVA would you try with this patient and why?

54 What forms of near correction are there and what are their advantages and disadvantages?

55 How can you tell what type of telescope this is? (Given a telescope)

56 How would you help a patient with RP for distance and near? What problems would they have with reading?

57 What problems would a patient with AMD have with reading? What sort of visual field defect are they likely to have? How could you help this patient?

58 How often would you see a patient after dispensing an LVA?

59 What is a BD8 and what happens to it?
60 Draw the ray diagrams for a Galilean, an astronomical telescope and a microscope stand magnifier.

10.6 MORE INFO?

Dickinson, C. *Low Vision: Principles and Practice.* Oxford: Butterworth-Heinemann, 1998.

Occupational optometry

Simon Brooks

11.1 WHAT DOES THE CO SAY?

The following information is taken from the CO pre-registration pack. The information in italics is my own and not provided by the CO. The syllabus is short and to the point: 'Environmental factors affecting visual efficiency. Regulation and statutory requirements.'

The GOC do not provide a specific core curriculum/core competencies for occupational optometry, but some information on standards can be found in the curriculum for Core Subject 4: Optical Appliances (find it in your pre-registration pack supplied by the CO). This will help you determine the standard you need to achieve in this subject.

The CO provide information under three headings: fitness to practise, nature of the examination and assessment.

Fitness to practise

'The qualified practitioner must be aware of the implications of the requirements for the performance of occupational and recreational visual task analysis *(VTA)*. He or she must be able to advise on and, where appropriate, supply appropriate appliances (possibly non-ophthalmic) and have a broad understanding of the characteristics of lighting and its effect on visual task performance.'

Nature of the examination

The examination comprises a 20-minute oral with two examiners. A range of relevant items will be available *(including safety glasses and lamps)*. Questions may be asked on any subject in the syllabus for this section. No patient will be provided.

Assessment

In each case the examiners will look to see that the candidate has:

(i)   Awareness of visual task analysis and specific visual requirements for various occupations.

(ii)   Understanding of the principles and methods of vision screening, and knowledge of advantages and disadvantages of such programmes for particular tasks.

(iii)   A knowledge of the factors that affect the visibility of a task and methods of improving visibility.

(iv)   A knowledge of:
   - the influence of illumination on (natural and artificial) upon visual performance
   - the use of colour and colour coding to improve visual performance and safety.

(v)   An understanding of the various light sources available, and their characteristics and suitability for various tasks.

(vi)   An awareness of levels of lighting required for particular tasks and the methods of measurement.

(vii)   An awareness of potential ocular hazards of various tasks and the consequences if the necessary eye protection is not provided.

(viii) A knowledge of responsibilities of the optometrist to a patient regarding the supply of eye protectors, the standards to which they are made and their identification.

11.2 THE EXAMINATION FORMAT

One of the examiners is likely to be a lighting engineer while the second will always be an optometrist. This exam does not involve a practical, but you may be shown lamps, eye protectors, photographs, or diagrams to identify and discuss. You will not need to take any equipment with you to this exam. Often the examination begins with an open-ended question that could relate to any aspect of the occupational optometry syllabus. It is a broad subject, incorporating important medico-legal considerations in parts of the syllabus. In this examination, candidates will need to show an understanding of the significance of a patient's occupation, hobbies and interests, and the considerations that should be made when prescribing optical appliances or offering advice to patients. Be prepared to be surprised! The selection of past questions at the end of this chapter will give you some idea of what to expect, but sometimes questions are vague. Remember that examiners do not want to give leading questions; the purpose of the exam is to determine what you know.

Towards the end of the examination, examiners may tire of asking questions and tend towards eccentricities. The visual requirements for Canadian

Mounted Police is not normally considered in a typical UK practice, yet this question has been asked. Do not be baffled by such questions. Try to think logically about the situation, e.g. the Canadian Mountie may be troubled by sun-glare, hence the uniform includes a wide-brimmed hat. The examiner may have a particular hobby or interest, e.g. cricket or painting, and you may be asked to consider the illumination and safety requirements for this type of task.

Initial questions tend to be less specific; you may be asked to describe the lighting arrangement in the examination room, in your place of work or in photographs you are shown. Examiners often ask about occupational considerations that you have made during the pre-registration year. It is therefore good preparation to discuss with your supervisor and fellow students when possible cases where eye protectors or special intermediate prescriptions have been advised or special colour vision assessments have been performed.

11.3 WHAT DO THE EXAMINERS SAY?

The following are comments provided by two examiners.

(a) What advice would you give to a candidate preparing for the exam?

   A: General advice for preparation includes reading relevant articles in the *Optician* journal, *OT* and other sources, and obtaining plenty of practical experience. If experience of occupational optometry is not forthcoming (this will almost certainly be the case for those students in the HES), then visits to private practices, factories and offices may help to increase awareness of ocular hazards and VTA.

   B: Awareness of lighting requirements and the use of colour coding may be improved by analysing these aspects during every visit to the supermarket, swimming pool, fitness centres, pub, and restaurant. Make careful note of unusual or innovative designs in your locality, and pay particular attention to lighting design and colour coding within the practice or hospital.

(b) What areas of the subject require

   (i)   Sound knowledge?

   A: Those aspects where the safety of the patient is paramount, e.g. eye protection and visual requirements for driving.

   B: Fundamental principles of lighting and illumination require attentive study, and although a lighting engineer will make allowances for the optometrist's lack of familiarity with some engineering terms, examiners are often amazed by candidates' lack of knowledge on this topic.

(ii)   Reasonable knowledge?
   A: The rest of the syllabus.
(iii) Some knowledge?
   A: Related topics, e.g. dispensing, LVA and emergency lighting, may be required. You will certainly need to know in detail the hazards of flicker and the stroboscopic effect, and how these problems are overcome.
(c) What do you look for in the successful candidate?
   A: The examiners are looking for candidates with a safe and confident approach, and with the ability to communicate effectively. They also hope to find a genuine interest in the subject, and this is where many candidates fail to impress!
(d) What brings people's marks down?
   A: An apparent indifference to the subject is due to candidates' inability to recognize its relevance. Consideration of illumination requirements and ocular safety is of vital importance in everyday practice. It should also be remembered that all the examiners in this subject have a keen interest in either occupational optometry or lighting design. A candidate who demonstrates an intelligent interest in the topic with a broad understanding of its basic principles, and who has the ability to utilize common sense, will do well.
(e) What are the common causes of failure?
   A: Indifferent performance, lack of preparation, and poor communication are the main causes of failure, especially where there is a danger to the public.

11.4 HELP AND ADVICE

Preparation for the exam

While working in your practice or hospital, maintain a constant awareness of VTA and illumination during the course of your normal working day. Try to visit two or three factories during the year. Remember that the occupational optometry PQE is in March or April. Obtain as much peripheral information as possible and keep aware of the changes in law. Attend meetings that include occupational optometry and lighting design modules. Sports Vision Association lectures will also be useful.

Revision! Those cups of coffee and tea and the king size bars of chocolate will once again be an important part of exam preparation! However, it may be necessary to change your approach to revision for these examinations. There are a number of differences between PQEs and the university exams. These differences may affect the way you go about your preparation. The main differences have been discussed elsewhere in this book, but here is a point to remember: you may not be able to cram until 5 am if your first appointment is at 9 am! Note that you no longer have the support network that university provides; lecture handouts, tutorials, library facilities, and fellow students. Because this is an oral exam it can take any direction and many subjects overlap, e.g. dispensing, low vision, BV, and drugs.

The scope of the exam

The CO syllabus gives a brief outline of the subjects examined, but it does not give a clear indication of the depth of knowledge that is required. The following list is not exhaustive, but is intended to demonstrate the level of expertise required, for each subject.

VTA

This is something that you will be doing during every eye examination when you ask about a patient's occupation and hobbies. You will then give consideration to their visual requirements during your examination and management. You will probably be doing everything correctly without actually realizing which parts of the routine eye examination have special relevance to this PQE. Generally, during a sight test allowances should be made for visibility of task and ergonomic factors; working distances, size and contrast of detail and whether stationary or moving; illumination, size of work area, hazards, danger, safety, degree of care or precision required, colour vision requirement, field of vision and stereopsis.

Consider a presbyopic patient. The final prescription issued, the type of spectacle frame(s) chosen and the decision for single vision lenses or multi-focals will all depend upon, and perhaps be limited by, occupational and recreational demands. Separate spectacles may be required for occupational and general use.

If the patient has a moving task then this will also influence your decision. A slowly moving target is likely to be followed by moving the whole head (this may cause problems with a 'swim' effect with varifocals). Whereas observation of a quickly moving near target will probably involve tracking (pursuit) eye movements and therefore a larger bifocal segment may be more appropriate.

Many occupations have specific visual requirements, and the more common of these are listed in the AOP handbook. However, you may be asked the visual requisites of an occupation that is not listed in the handbook; the candidate will be expected to show initiative and common sense, while demonstrating safety and competence.

The standard requirement for driving is in the AOP handbook, along with requirements for different types of vehicles. The candidate needs to understand how to determine these standards in the practice and what action to take if a patient fails to meet a standard. This depends on the circumstances of course, but may involve a referral either to the GP or to an ophthalmologist. Candidates are sometimes asked whether they would contact the DVLA if a patient persists in driving with sub-standard vision. This presents a dilemma between two ethical responsibilities: patient confidentiality and duty of care, first and foremost to the patient and second to the public.

Many people now use visual display units (VDUs) at home and work, so it is important to ask about VDU use during the eye examination. Do not assume that certain people do not use computers; you will often be surprised. The *Health and Safety (Display Screen Equipment – DSE) Regulations 1992* followed a European Directive in 1990, and aims to protect the DSE user. It considers workstation analysis, daily work routines, eyes and sight testing, provision of corrective appliances, training, and health and safety information. These regulations have been in effect since 1993. Optometrists should be aware of all sections of these regulations, because although the section on sight testing has the most relevance, ergonomic factors, work schedules and adequate training will have some influence on patients' perceived comfort. Postural ischaemia causes many problems, including symptoms such as eyestrain.

Employees who are about to become users are entitled to an eye examination on request, as are those who are already DSE users. Employees may opt for vision screening if available, without jeopardizing the right to a full assessment if this becomes necessary. Prescriptions should be issued to the employees and details of examination are only issued to the employer with the patient's consent.

It is important to understand the characteristics of DSE that can cause eyestrain: character dimensions, luminance of display and background luminance, flicker, jitter and refresh rate. Colours displayed may cause focusing problems, particularly if two colours at opposite ends of the spectrum are displayed on the screen simultaneously. Reflections off the screen may cause glare, which can be reduced or eliminated by using an anti-glare screen, such as mesh, polarized, notched or neutral density anti-reflection coated plastic. UV radiation is minimal; less than a colour TV. Epileptogenic factors are possible but susceptible individuals would have similar problems with TV. Remember the effects of fatigue, due to accumulation of lactic acid in the ciliary body, and a reduction in normal blink rate in DSE users.

Vision screening

The principle is to have a set of requirements that a patient will pass or fail! If the subject fails then referral for a full eye examination follows. Any test such as this will have a small percentage of false positives and false negatives. Understand what is meant by the terms specificity and sensitivity. The added complication here is that the test/pass requirement differs with the optometrist's criteria. There is a risk of false positives having undiagnosed pathology and not seeking an optometrist's advice, unaware of any problem.

The accuracy of these instruments may be affected by proximal accommodation and convergence. Candidates may be required to recognize a vision screener, be able to evaluate it and show how it is used.

Illumination

Be familiar with the definitions and units of the following: luminous flux (lm), luminous efficacy (lmW^{-1}), luminance (cdm^{-2}), illuminance (lmm^{-2}) and luminous intensity (cd), vector/scalar ratio. The inverse square law describes the relationship between the illuminance on a surface and its distance from the light source. Patients who are struggling to read in artificial light will benefit from using a desk or table lamp with an adjustable arm. However, the effect of improved illumination, whether by changing light source or its distance from the task, is subject to the law of diminishing returns, i.e. the illumination eventually saturates and visual performance remains the same even if the illumination is further increased. The illumination at which performance plateaus is dependent upon the task. It should be appreciated that in certain circumstances it will be easier to improve the visibility of a task by changing a parameter other than illumination, e.g. size of detail or working distance.

Visibility may also be improved by utilizing colour. Colour coding may be connotative where the colour conveys a precise message, or denotative where the colour is redundant because the message is conveyed by other means, but the coding helps to speed up response. About eight per cent of the male population is colour deficient. There are a number of types of deficiencies and many colour vision tests. It is important to know these well and some knowledge of Committee International d'Eclairage (CIE) Specification of Chromaticity (1931) is useful. Because colour coding plays such an important role in safety and awareness of hazards, many occupations demand a specific degree of colour discrimination. Certain colour codes are safe for all, e.g. the domestic electrical wiring code and gaseous anaesthetics in medicine. The traffic light code is only safe for all because it is sequenced. Often luminance contrast is utilized in conjunction with colour contrast. Where there is a high-risk hazard flashing lights and audio cues may also be used.

Lighting

One examiner commented 'It is surprising how little is known about lamps and how to use them'. It is important to understand the principles of black body radiation and colour temperature, incandescence and how incandescent lamps have evolved. The candidate will also need to understand how gas discharge lamps and fluorescent lamps work and the way these differ from incandescent light sources, in construction, operation and cost to run, luminous efficacy, colour rendering properties, and CCT class. It's all in the Chartered Institution of Building Services Engineers (CIBSE) reference text.

The effects of oscillation with discharge and fluorescent light sources, due to AC electrical supply are important to remember. Usually the oscillation is faster than the critical flicker frequency of the eye and is therefore invisible. This invisible oscillation affects the appearance of revolving equipment. This is called the stroboscopic effect and it is a serious hazard in industry; revolving propellers could, in certain conditions, appear stationary! You will need to know how this problem is overcome in industry. Occasionally, flicker may become visible, e.g. towards the end of the lamp life. Visible flicker is annoying and may reduce productivity. It is a possible cause of migraine attacks and epileptic fits. Even invisible flicker may have a subliminal effect in certain individuals.

Sound knowledge is required of various types of luminaire and their characteristics with respect to protection from impact, water, fire and such like, mounting position, polar curve distribution, and the various ergonomic and commercial factors that influence their design. Light is controlled either by obstruction, diffusion, refraction or reflection.

Optometrists are concerned with lighting for two main reasons. First, poor lighting may affect the comfort and efficiency of our patient and cause symptoms. Second, refined lighting design may improve visual comfort and productivity. To ensure the provision of appropriate advice, an understanding of the principles employed by the lighting engineer is necessary. The whole procedure is quite involved and it is not necessary to learn all the details, but knowledge of the CIBSE to acquire a basic understanding would be useful. The engineer first has a set of objectives for which a specification of compatible design criteria is determined. General planning involving assessment of the daylight factor, choices of lamps and luminaires then follows. Detailed planning includes assessment of costs, the utilization factor, the room index and light loss factors, reflectances, calculation of illuminance at task, and glare index. Finally, appraisal should include subjective assessment by the designer, photometric surveys, and discussions with the client and user.

Requirements and measurements of lighting levels

This information is readily available in CIBSE, which lists the standard service illuminance and limiting glare index for numerous activities and tasks encountered in various occupations. It is good preparation to know the lighting requirements of a number of tasks more commonly experienced in optometric practice. In the exam you may be required to estimate the required illuminance of a rather obscure task. You should give a considered estimate and explain the reasons for this requirement, which will include the visual demands and duration, the visual capability of the person performing the task and the degree of care involved. Knowledge is required of illuminance meters, which usually consist of silicon or selenium photovoltaic cells and luminance meters, which may be photovoltaic cells or photo multiplier tubes.

Protection

Certain occupations and activities present hazards to the eyes. These fall into three main categories: mechanical, chemical and radiation.

Mechanical

Dust causes irritation that depends on the substance. The trauma caused by impact will depend on the type of object involved, e.g. sharp or blunt, hard or soft. Small fast-moving projectiles are more likely to penetrate the cornea than larger objects, which tend to cause crushing or lacerating injuries. A splash of molten metal causes mechanical injury heat damage and may be toxic, e.g. copper.

Chemical splashes and noxious vapours

Effects will be different for acids, alkalis and bleaches; alkali splashes tend to be more serious than acid because they penetrate human tissue more deeply. Systemically ingested poisons may produce symptoms.

Radiation

Background X-rays present little hazard to the eye. Ultra-violet from the sun, or from various other sources, e.g. welding, dental and printing equipment, may cause transient damage such as 'arc eye', or more long-term problems such as cataract formation. Different wavelengths within the ultra-violet range present different levels of hazard and it is important to understand these differences. Light of sufficient intensity may also present a hazard to the eye, although the damage caused will probably be due to heat. Lasers are restricted to a safety limit of 3 mVm^{-2}. Long-term exposure to infrared radiation, e.g. in steel or glass industries can cause a characteristic posterior cataract. Microwaves from radar, telecommunications and industrial ovens have an unofficial safety limit of 100 Wm^{-2}. Domestic microwave ovens have a leakage limit of 10 Wm^{-2}. It is particularly important to consider that eye injuries do not occur in industry alone. Most occur outside the workplace during leisure activities, such as sports, DIY and gardening.

The general principle of protection is to shield the source of hazard and then the individual at risk. The type of protector is dependent on the type of hazard and may include spectacles with robust frames, moulded eye shields, face shields, box and cup type goggles, and welding helmets and shields. Materials are polycarbonate, CR39, PMMA, toughened glass, and laminated glass.

It is important to have a working knowledge of the regulations introduced under the Health and Safety at Work Act 1974: The Management of Health and Safety at Work Regulations 1992; The Personal Protective Equipment at Work

Regulations 1992; The Workplace (Health, Safety and Welfare) Regulations 1992; The Provision and Use of Work Equipment Regulations 1992; The Health and Safety Display Screen Equipment Regulations 1992; The Manual Handling Operations Regulations 1992.

It would be useful to have a working knowledge of the following European standards for eye protection: BS EN 165 Personal Eye Protection–Vocabulary; BS EN 166 Personal Eye Protection–Specifications; BS EN 167 Personal Eye Protection–Optical Test Methods; BS EN 168 Personal Eye Protection–Non-optical Test Methods; BS EN 168 Personal Eye Protection–Filters for Welding and Similar Operations; BS EN 170 Personal Eye Protection–Ultra-violet Light Filters; BS EN 171 Personal Eye Protection–Infra-red Filters; BS EN 172 Personal Eye Protection–Sun Glare Filters; BS EN 175 Personal Eye Protection–Equipment for Eye and Face Protection During Welding and Allied Processes; BS EN 207 Personal Eye Protection–Filters and Eye-Protectors Against Laser Radiation; BS EN 379 Personal Eye Protection–Welding Filters With Switchable Luminous Transmittance and With Dual Luminous Transmittance.

More details can be found in the text by North, see the More Info? section.

Responsibilities of the optometrist

Although the industrial safety officer will often organize the type of eye protector to be issued to an employee, it is ultimately the responsibility of the optometrist to ensure that the appliance is appropriate and is manufactured to the approved specification.

This requires sound knowledge of the relevant legislation and the relevant BS EN documents. Incorrect use of an appliance, or an appliance that is below standard, may have devastating consequences for the user and could lead to litigation. If an appliance is made to an approved specification suitable for the task for which it is to be used, then should injury occur the optometrist could not be deemed to be at fault. An appliance made to a BS EN standard will be marked accordingly. The marking of the appliance and methods of testing so that it meets the standard required is set out in the relevant European Standard specification.

11.5 PAST EXAM QUESTIONS

1 If you had to design lighting for a hospital, what would you have to consider and what levels of illumination are required?
2 What are the properties of polycarbonate lenses as opposed to CR39 lenses?
3 What is colour coding? Give an example of its use.
4 What type of lighting is used in this exam room? What lux is it?

5 What levels of lighting are necessary for the following:
   (a) An office
   (b) A library
   (c) A squash court
   (d) A living room
   (e) The cockpit of an airplane?
6 What visual requirements must a pilot satisfy (a) in civil operations, (b) in the armed forces
7 What happens if a halogen bulb is touched?
8 What type of lighting is used for the following:
   (a) Street lights
   (b) Security and exit lights
   (c) Shop window lights
   (d) Football stadium
   (e) Car headlights?
9 Have you ever had a patient with a sport/hobby/occupation-related eye condition? What eye protection were they wearing? What should they wear?
10 What does VTA stand for? How many times have you carried out a VTA?
11 Here is an electronic circuit board. What are the visual requirements for its assembly? What are the coloured bands on the smaller components for?
12 How can you calculate near visual acuity requirement?
13 What is the X-ray warning sign? What is the laser warning sign? What is laser an acronym for?
14 What type of lamp is this? What problems may occur in its use? What substance is the envelope made from?
15 Which body gives information on required lighting levels?
16 What are the differences between a filament GLS (general light source) and a compact fluorescent tube?
17 What is the visual standard required for driving? Does it take into account visual fields? What field defect is most dangerous? Does it matter if you only have one eye?
18 What types of high-pressure discharge lamps are available? At what frequency does flicker occur with discharge lamps? Does flicker vary with the distance along a fluorescent tube? How can you avoid this? Is flicker dangerous?
19 What are the principles of street lighting? Why use sodium lamps?
20 Discuss lighting in a swimming pool. What sort of problems with glare would you have in a swimming pool? What types of glare are there?
21 Have you dispensed protective eyewear? What approved specification did it conform to? How did you know it conformed to this?
22 How would you find the standard of vision required for a given occupation? What would you do if the occupation is not listed?

23 Define luminance and illuminance. How are they measured?

24 In what way has BS 2092 been changed recently (1988)?

25 If a patient has an accident while wearing eye protection supplied by you, how might you stand legally if the appliance was (a) kite marked, (b) not kite marked but in accordance with appropriate specification, (c) kite marked but to a specification inappropriate for the task?

26 Can you reglaze or repair a protective spectacle frame that was made to British Standards?

27 What is a vision screener and what is it used for?

28 A photographer has the spectacle prescription $R + 1.25 / - 0.50 \times 70$, $L + 1.75 / - 0.75 \times 90$ and he has trouble focusing the camera. What would you advise?

29 What problems might the user of a VDU encounter?

30 What obligations lie with the employer if VDUs are used?

31 A patient has the following spectacle prescription $R + 2.50 / - 2.00 \times 180$, $L + 5.75 / - 3.00 \times 160$. Are there likely to be any problems if the patient wants to be a research chemist?

32 You are shown a photograph of a painter painting a white outside wall. What are the visual problems? How can they be reduced? Is protective eyewear required?

33 What sort of lighting do you have in your practice? Why is this sort used? What is the normal level for consulting room lighting? What is the British Standard illuminance of a test chart?

34 What are the main groups of ocular hazard for which protective eyewear caters?

35 What is the principle of motorway and roundabout lighting?

36 What are the advantages of small compact fluorescent tubes for use in the home?

37 What type of eye protector is this? Explain the markings. For what sort of task would this protector be used?

38 Why doesn't the visual requirement for driving correspond exactly to Snellen acuity?

39 How would the appearance of the optic disc vary with different types of ophthalmoscope bulb? What types of bulb are commonly used in ophthalmic instruments?

40 What is the minimum illuminance in which the eye can function?

41 At what level of illuminance would cricket stop play?

42 Would you prescribe varifocals for someone who regularly uses a lathe? What sort of lighting would you advise?

43 What tasks in the home and in the garden require eye protection?

44 What is the standard specification for protective eyewear for welding tasks? What markings would you expect? What does GWF stand for?

45 Does cleaning a polycarbonate lens with acetone have any effect on the material?

46 You are shown the photograph of a policeman wearing a yellow jacket with white stripes. What are the stripes for? Why is the jacket yellow? What is fluorescence?

47 When a person goes fishing, what sort of problems might she experience? What sort of glasses would you recommend?

48 What sort of lamp is this? What is its efficacy and what is its life? What are its other characteristics?

49 What are the AOP recommendations for VDU users and what do you think of them?

50 Would you recommend contact lenses for someone who is a:
   (a) Welder
   (b) Squash player
   (c) Cricketer
   (d) Research chemist
   (e) Swimmer
   (f) VDU operator
   (g) Cook?

51 What is the lumen method of lighting design?

52 What are the recommended levels of illuminance for (a) a vision chart (vertical plane), (b) an operating theatre cavity?

53 Give a summary of what is outlined in BS EN 166.

54 What is the vision requirement for personal car use?

55 What is the driving standard for a taxi driver?

56 What occupations require normal colour vision?

57 Compare and contrast tungsten and fluorescent lighting.

58 What is colour rendering?

59 What are the ocular effects of ultra-violet radiation?

60 What is connotative colour rendering?

11.6 MORE INFO?

North, R. *Work and the Eye*, second edition. Oxford: Butterworth-Heinemann, 2000.

Smith, NA. *Lighting for Occupational Optometry* (HHSC Handbook Series). Safchem Services, 1999.

CIBSE Code for Interior Lighting, revised edition. The Chartered Institution of Building Services Engineers, 1998. Delta House, 222 Balham High Road, London SW11 9BF.

12

Dispensing

Janet Carlton, Frank Eperjesi and Alicia Thompson

12.1 WHAT DOES THE CO SAY?

The GOC do not provide a specific core curriculum/core competencies for dispensing but some information on standards can be found in the curriculum for Core Subject 4: Optical Appliances (find it on the CD in your pre-registration pack supplied by the CO). This will help you determine the standard you need to achieve in this subject.

Fitness to practise

'During the prescribing of a new optical appliance the practitioner is required to take full account of a patient's previous prescription, which must be precisely neutralized.

An analysis of the new prescription and the patient's needs will precede a discussion on alternative and preferred ways of dispensing, in the light of knowledge about ophthalmic frames and lenses.'

Nature of the examination

Practical

This part of the examination is in the form of a station examination. The candidate will be expected to perform seven different tasks each of which will be allocated ten minutes. At the end of each ten-minute period, the candidate will be required to move to the next task allocated to him/her.

Oral

This part of the examination will last for 30 minutes and will be with two examiners. When the oral follows the station examination, it may commence with the candidate being asked to discuss the results of the tasks performed during the station examination. This will then be extended to a general discussion on lens and frame materials, methods of manufacture, lens designs and their advantages and disadvantages, and British Standards relating to frames and lenses. When the oral precedes the station examination, it will take the form of a general oral and may include hypothetical examples. Candidates will be expected to write out a prescription order, which will be discussed. A lens catalogue (Norville) will be provided.

Assessment

The candidate will be expected to:

(i)   Identify and quantify parameters of spectacle lenses and frames that would be required to enable an exact duplicate to be ordered.
(ii) Analyse a prescription and discuss sensibly the alternative and preferred methods of dispensing.
(iii) Write a final order for a pair of spectacles that allows the prescription house to process it as intended, without query.
(iv) Demonstrate an understanding of the optical principles underlying current ophthalmic lens/frame design and production.

12.2 WHAT DO THE EXAMINERS SAY?

Examiners in dispensing provided the following information.

(a) What advice would you give to a candidate preparing for the exam?
     A: It is essential for the candidate to demonstrate practical dispensing knowledge. The characteristics of all the lenses that they have dispensed, their advantages and disadvantages, must be known.
     B: Read around the subject and not only lecture notes.
     C: The examiners are primarily looking for fitness to practise. The public expects and deserves sound and informed advice from a qualified optician about spectacles and optical appliances.
     D: The candidate must ensure that during the PQE year they have ordered, verified and fitted a variety of frames and lens types. They should read all new literature supplied by the optical companies and should regularly read the dispensing articles in the *Optician* and *OT* publications.
(b) What areas of the subject require:
     (i)   Sound knowledge?
           A: Safety lenses and frames.
           B: Lens materials, multifocal fitting, spectacle frame fitting and adjustments.
           C: The suitability of lens and frame types for certain cases. The relative advantages and disadvantages of available alternatives.

Knowledge of correct fitting of frames and lenses, especially multifocals.

D: Knowledge of lens design and application. Knowledge of frame materials and their limitations. An ability to recognize and discuss the properties of different lens and frame designs. An ability to solve simple mathematical problems involving the prismatic effect.

(ii) Reasonable knowledge?

B: Frame materials.

C: Knowledge of currently available materials and designs, of lenses and frames in general terms.

D: Tints and their application. The problems of UV and possible pathological effects of over exposure.

(iii) Some knowledge?

B: Frame and lens manufacture.

C: Specific product knowledge, particularly where certain products are unique to certain manufacturers. Knowledge of materials and designs not currently used but which might be encountered on the odd occasion, e.g. frame materials such as nitrate or real shell.

D: Transmission curves. Light transmission through materials of different refractive index.

(c) What do you look for in the successful candidate?

A: Rational thinking, e.g. 'What lenses would you prescribe for a skier?' requires an answer including safety and UV protection.

B: Candidates should have a basically sound knowledge of the subject and demonstrate that they are fit to practise.

C: Familiarity with frames and lenses. Some candidates react as though they have never handled spectacles before. An ability to show that they know what the best options are for their patients and why they are the best options. Confidence in their own knowledge with the ability to answer questions on fundamental practical issues such as simple interpretation of a given prescription.

(d) What brings people's marks down?

A: Poor knowledge of frames and lenses, especially if the lens in question is one used by the candidate.

B: Making statements with confidence that are demonstrably flawed and being unable to explain concepts in a clear concise way, as might be required by an enquiring patient.

C: Taking too long to answer questions. Not appreciating what's important, e.g. if asked about AR coatings some candidates will talk about quarter wavelengths, square roots of refractive indices, half waves out of step and such like, without ever mentioning the reduction of reflections!

D: A totally inaccurate answer. An inability to explain clearly and concisely a point and thereby allow only a few questions to be asked in the time allowed for the oral.

(e) What are the common causes of failure?

A: Failure to spot a possible non-tolerance factor in a prescription, e.g. vertical prism imbalance.

B: Not showing a basic understanding of the subject.

C: Candidates will fail if they show a general lack of knowledge in most of the areas they are questioned on. Candidates who have obviously not studied enough and have not prepared properly will be failed.

D: Some candidates have an obvious lack of interest in this subject and this comes through during the oral. Little or no background reading. A poor grasp of the most basic concepts of understanding frame and lens design, manufacture and use.

(f) What subject areas do candidates place too little importance upon?

A: Many candidates give me the impression that dispensing is beneath them and do no serious studying or preparation. Reading through university notes is not enough.

B: Familiarity of common aspects of progressive and aspheric lenses and the use of tints. Candidates should strive to keep up to date with lens availability in general.

C: Fundamental principles of ophthalmic lenses seem to be forgotten about by the time the PQEs come along.

D: Following the routine examination during the pre-registration year, very few candidates pay attention to blank size, lens thickness and prismatic effect when the glasses are ordered from the lens laboratory. In order to gain understanding of the possible problems, this type of analysis should be done regularly.

(g) Any other comments?

D: Some candidates treat dispensing lightly because it is not an 'academic' subject. They fail to realize the true depth of modern knowledge and often do not appreciate the importance of this subject in the practice. As a result many are poorly prepared for the exam.

12.3 PREPARATION ADVICE

During your pre-registration year, try to dispense, fit, check, and adjust as many types of lenses and frames as possible. Do not shy away from difficult dispensings but always have your work checked and critically analysed by the dispensing optician or your supervisor. Read all lens and frame suppliers' promotional literature and become familiar with different types of design with the same lens type, e.g. progressives. Read the frequent dispensing articles published in the *Optician* and *OT*. Arrange to visit the closest lens manufacturing facility to gain a better insight into lens and coating production.

Practical exam advice

The examination paper will be sent to you by the CO. Study it carefully and go over it with your supervisor, make sure you understand every word and practise each task regularly prior to taking the exam. Ask your supervisor to time, mark and critically analyse your work. There are ten minutes for each of the practical stations. During the exam you should only have to check which station you are at, take a few seconds to remind yourself of what you have to do and then get started. Read the question carefully and write your answers clearly. Give sufficient and relevant information, i.e. do not measure the right lens if the left has been asked for.

Look at the equipment list. This will give a clue as to what is required but remember that just because a particular piece of equipment is available doesn't mean that you have to use it. When using the focimeter always zero it and adjust the eyepiece for yourself. Zero the prism compensator if there is one present. Check that the lens measure reads zero on a flat surface and familiarize yourself with which scale is positive and which is negative.

General tolerances are $+/-0.25$ D in sphere, cylinder and addition, $+/-5$ degrees in axis, $+/-2$ mm in centration, $+/-0.5$ prism dioptres. However, errors in measurements are assessed as an outcome to the wearer so 90 degrees off-axis, for example, will result in zero for that lens.

The stations

Station 1

Using the equipment provided, record the lens details and full specifications of the **LEFT** *lens provided.*

This station requires you to write down everything about the lens supplied so that the lab can produce a duplicate. This is usually a varifocal lens, the engravings are made obvious and appropriate templates are supplied. A routine for this station may be: sphere, cylinder, axis, addition, prism at the ref. point, material, tint, horizontal monocular centres, fitting cross height, form, i.e sphere curve of lens ($F1$ – note on varifocal; this is taken horizontally with centre leg on prism reference point).

Station 2

Using the equipment provided, record (a) the refractive index and (b) the true surface powers of the **LEFT** *lens of the spectacles provided.*

Usually the lens to be measured has been made in plano-concave form but check using the 'straight-edge test' or lens measure.

(a) Refractive index

$$\frac{0.523 \times F\ (\text{actual})}{F\ (\text{lens measure})} = (n-1)\ \text{actual}$$

Check that your answer makes sense! Plastics indices range from 1.498–1.74 and glass range from 1.523–1.9.

(b) True surface powers
The curve variation factor (*CVF*) will need to be calculated, using the curve variation equation:

$$\frac{0.523}{F\ (\text{lens measure})} = \frac{n\ (\text{actual})-1}{0.523}$$

Multiplying the CVF by the value found for each lens surface gives the true surface power of the lens:

$$CVF \times F\ (\text{lens measure}) = \text{true surface power}$$

However if *F1* is flat the surface is plano, whatever the index.

If you are presented with a toric lens, you will have two focimeter readings and two lens measure readings for *F2*. You only need one pair of readings but ensure you take corresponding meridians. If a plus lens is supplied the situation becomes more complex. The following equation will replace $F1 + F2 = F'v$:

$$F'v = \frac{F1 + F2 - dF1F2}{1 - dF2}$$

where $d = t/n$, *t* is measured in metres using thickness callipers and $n = 1.523$.

Station 3

Using the equipment provided, record the listed frame measurements of the frame provided.

This station requires plenty of practice. To prepare, make sure you have a frame rule. Then sort out 20 frames and spend time each day measuring them. Write down the results so when the same frame is measured at a later date the answers can be checked. You will need to know how to measure the following: boxed lens size and distance between lenses, bridge height, bridge width, frontal angle, joint height, bridge projection, downward angle of drop, head width, splay angle of pad, temple width, angle of side. Tolerances for measurements are +/−1 mm, for angles +/−5 degrees, and +/−5 mm tolerance is allowed on temple/head width and length to bend. Mistakes will result in negative marking. Do not attempt to adjust the frame under any circumstances.

Station 4

Using the equipment provided, record the listed facial measurements of the patient.

This station requires plenty of previous practice. For practising, make sure you have a facial rule with the instruction booklets. Find suitable volunteers in your practice and measure them on a weekly basis. Make sure you are taking the measurements properly. If in doubt ask your supervisor or the practice dispensing optician for advice or to check your measurements. You will need to know the following: pupillary distance and near centration distance (may be measured using a frame rule), head width, distance between rims at 10 mm below crest, distance between rims at 15 mm below crest, frontal angle, splay angle, projection, apical radius, angle of crest, crest/bridge height. Tolerances for measurements are $+/-2$ mm, for angles $+/-5$ degrees, while $+/-5$ mm tolerance is allowed on head width and length to bend. Mistakes will result in negative marking.

Station 5

Using the equipment provided, adjust the frame to fit the patient.

The only way to become skilled at frame adjustment is to practise constantly throughout the pre-registration year. Try and do as many collections and adjustments as possible.

First, assess the set-up of the frame on the bench – check the front isn't twisted and the let-back equal to both sides. Sit the frame on the bench with ear-points facing down, adjust angle of side to correct rocking. Then assess fit on the face, using the 'fitting triangle'. Start with the bridge fitting/pad alignment, and then look at the plane of front and pantoscopic tilt. Next look at temple/head width and length to bend, and then check the downward and inward angle of drop. Check set-up and closure symmetry, and finally clean the spectacles. Note: the method of adjustment is not marked, only the final result. If a breakage occurs, another frame will be given but no extra time.

Station 6

Using the equipment provided, record the specification of the spectacles at the box centre position.

The main function of this station is to assess your ability to measure prism using the focimeter. In this station, just because there is a trial case doesn't mean that it has to be used. If the focimeter provided has a prism compensator, check that it is zeroed with the dioptre scale at zero and the base scale at 90.

First, accurately mark the boxed centre and then measure sphere, cylinder and axis. Next measure the prism to 0.25 D and the base direction.

Make sure you measure both lenses. If the focimeter is unfamiliar, use a trial prism to check the scale. If prism in the spectacles is very large, use a trial prism or prism-compensator to bring the image back into view and add in the neutralizing prism to obtain the overall value.

Station 7

Using the equipment provided, verify the specification of the LEFT LENS AND FRAME of the spectacles supplied and note any errors.

The candidate should check as many orders as possible during the pre-registration year. The following is a checking routine you might consider useful: prescription details, frame details, lens material, type of lens, tint correct, coating correct, size, shape and height of bifocals, centration details (including inset), prism, glazing faults.

Be very clear on error versus order, i.e. 'right axis is 90 degrees, should be 180'. Marks are awarded for noting the error and measuring it correctly.

Oral exam advice

The oral examination will last 30 minutes with two examiners. The list below gives an indication of broad subjects covered but is by no means the complete syllabus. Example questions are also given in the next section.

- Tasks performed in the stations may be discussed in more detail in the oral.
- Demonstrate knowledge of relevant BS and EN Standards relating to spectacle frames, lenses and personal eye protection.
- You may be asked to write out a final order so that the prescription house can produce a pair of spectacles without reference or query.
- You are very likely to be asked to interpret a given prescription and offer sound and reasoned dispensing advice, offering solutions to possible problems.
- Demonstrate a sound knowledge of current lens designs, i.e. aspheric, lenticular and best form.
- Lens materials and their properties, i.e. polycarbonate, high index,
- Lens applications, methods of manufacture and principles.
- How facial and frame measurements relate and consequences of alteration.
- Identification of frame materials, properties and methods of manufacture.
- Prisms – use of, surfaced, decentred, slab-off, prism thinning, prism-controlled.
- Lens availability – single vision, bifocals, trifocals, varifocals, occupational lenses.

- Estimation of power of a given lens.
- Calculation of minimum size uncut using a ruler, given frame and pupillary distance.
- Explanation of blanksize, importance for plus and minus prescriptions.
- Know your own spectacles – lens and frame material and method of manufacture!

12.4 PAST EXAM QUESTIONS

1 What is the difference between gold filled and rolled gold?
2 Can titanium frames be repaired?
3 Name three frames with reinforcement in the sides.
4 Name three frames without reinforcement in the sides.
5 How would you differentiate between two solid black frames, one made of cellulose nitrate and one of cellulose acetate?
6 This prescription R − 1.00 DS, L − 5.00 DS is to be glazed into a rimless mount, in CR39, eye size 52 mm with no decentration. Centre substance of the L stock lens is 1 mm. What centre thickness does the R lens need to have to give equal edge thickness?
7 Find the different prismatic effects of the following lenses:
   (a) R +2.00 DS L +4.00 DS
   (b) R −2.00/−3.00 × 90 L −2.00/−3.00 × 90
   (c) R +2.00/+2.00 × 90 L +2.00/+3.00 × 135
8 Which measurements need to be taken to dispense the following prescription, R − 3.00/−0.75 × 90 L − 3.00 DS Add + 1.50 for (a) bifocals (b) varifocals?
9 Give three practical solutions for the dispensing of the following prescription, R − 6.00 DS, L − 4.00 DS Add + 2.00.
10 When would you recommend and how should you fit a 38 seg bifocal?
11 Why are executive bifocals optically poor?
12 Which are better: glass fused or glass solid bifocals? What are the advantages and disadvantages of each?
13 Would varifocals be useful for the following patients:
   (a) First-time presbyope
   (b) First-time varifocal wearer with + 3.00 DS add
   (c) A carpenter
   (d) An emmetropic presbyope VDU user
   (e) A patient needing a large near area
   (f) Patient with prescription R − 1.00 DS, L − 3.00 DS Add + 1.50
   (g) A patient with arthritis?
14 Where are the optical centres in a bifocal lens?
15 What advice would you give to a golfer who needs both distance and near correction?
16 What advice would you give on eye protection to someone who skis?

17 How would you reduce the head width on an acetate frame?

18 What properties does Optyl have?

19 When would you consider using a prism controlled bifocal?

20 What are the different types of prism control?

21 How is an acetate frame made and how are different colourings achieved?

22 What options are available to dispense a -8.00 DS prescription?

23 What principles are AR coats based upon? How is an AR coat applied to a lens? How is a hard coat applied?

24 Tell me about photochromics

25 Given the following prescription R $+2.00$ DS, L $+2.00/+3.00 \times 180$ Add $+2.00$ DS, what is the prism at 10 mm below optical centre?

26 How would you manage such a patient?

27 How can you correct anisometropia with a varifocal?

28 What progressive lenses do you use and why?

29 You are given the examiner's glasses and asked what prescription are these?

30 Discuss this tortoise-shell frame.

31 You are given cosmetic frames (make-up specs) and asked what it is?

32 What are Fresnel lenses and what are they used for?

33 Tell me about toughened prescription lenses and their relative merits.

34 Can you use grade 1 polycarbonate for prescription purposes?

35 Does a chip in a chemical or heat toughened lens affect its impact resistance?

36 Can any lens be heat toughened?

37 What frame and lens materials would you use for a child?

38 What is Trivex?

39 Name some plastic frame materials

40 Can an unregistered optician dispense glasses to a child?

41 What problems arise with nylon frames?

42 Would you use glass lenses in a child's frame?

43 Which is best, heat or chemical toughened?

44 Draw an upcurve bifocal

45 Can you make a full-face frame from acrylic?

46 Have you dispensed a supra frame?

47 Do you know what epoxy resin is?

48 Can you mend a broken aluminium frame?

49 What does 1/10 12K mean when stamped on a frame?

50 What do thermosetting and thermoplastic mean? Do these terms apply to lens or frame materials or both?

51 Name some materials that are thermosetting and some that are thermoplastic

52 What do you consider to be the advantages of varifocal lenses?

53 What do you consider to be the disadvantages of varifocal lenses?

54 What do you consider to be the disadvantages of bifocals?

55 What type of frame would you advise for a patient who has good distance vision, who needs single vision near lenses but also has a distance vision task?

56 What measurements are required when dispensing varifocal lenses?

57 Are there any performance differences between flat top and round bifocal segments?

58 What is a Franklin split bifocal and when might it prove useful?

59 How are prisms made?

60 How are plastic lenses tinted?

12.5 MORE INFO?

Fowler, CW and Latham, K. *Spectacle Lenses: Theory and Practice*. Oxford: Butterworth Heinemann, 2001.

Jalie, M. *Ophthalmic Lenses and Dispensing*, second edition. Oxford: Butterworth-Heinemann, 2003.

Bennett's Ophthalmic Prescription Work, fourth edition. Oxford: Butterworth-Heinemann, 2000.

Relevant European Standards, legislation and guidance. Make sure you keep up with recent revisions and additions!

13

Routine examination

John O'Donnell

The Routine PQE may look at first glance like an examination that is impossible to revise for. Although there is an element of truth to this, there are many things that you can do to prepare for this PQE.

13.1 WHAT THE CO SAYS

The following information is taken from the CO pre-registration pack. The information in italics is my own and not provided by the CO. The syllabus is short and to the point: 'The routine optometric examination of a patient'. *Well actually, two patients.*

The GOC do not provide specific core curriculum/core competencies for routine examination but some information on standards can be found in the curriculum for Core Subject 3: Refractive Management (find it in your pre-registration pack supplied by the CO). This will help you determine the standard you need to achieve in this subject.

The CO provide information under three headings: fitness to practise, nature of the examination and assessment.

Fitness to practise

'The object of the eye examination must be to ensure the optimum visual efficiency of the patient. To achieve this the Optometrist must understand the patient's symptoms and history and carry out the necessary tests related to them. The examination MUST ensure the detection of presenting pathology and must establish the visual status of the patient. From all the information produced by the examination, the Optometrist must arrive at an appropriate conclusion in the form of prescription, referral and advice or further examination. Candidates in the PQE must prove that they are capable of doing this safely.'

Nature of the examination

'The candidate is required to examine two patients. There will be two examiners and each will observe a complete routine examination of a patient by the candidate. One patient will be presbyopic and one pre-presbyopic. The time of 45 minutes will be allocated for the examination of each patient. The examiner for the first patient may indicate on the mark sheet any weak points that need to be assessed by the second examiner.

Once the candidate has examined both the presbyopic and pre-presbyopic patients there will be a ten-minute oral with both examiners. In the oral, questions may be asked on any part of the syllabus for this section.

Good patient handling and a safe, adequate routine are expected. The candidate may be asked to discuss any need for further attention, referral, prognosis, and patient management in the oral based on the completed records.

When a patient has spectacles these will NOT be made available to the candidate. The examination of each patient should comprise all those tests and assessments considered to be necessary by the candidate given the presenting signs and symptoms and the patient's history.'

Assessment

'The examiners will look to see that the candidate has:

(i)   Completed each procedure in the examination in a smooth and logical order.

(ii)   Demonstrated a command of techniques adequate to produce accurate results and an ability to demonstrate alternative techniques if necessary.

(iii)   Achieved a reasonable degree of accuracy throughout – in particular retinoscopy must be within 1 DS–1 DC and the axis orientation appropriately accurate to the amount of cylindrical correction.

(iv)   Not failed to recognize significant findings.

(v)   Shown themselves capable of establishing a professional relationship and that they are in control of the examination.

(vi)   Demonstrated a clear understanding of the results they achieve.

(vii)   Made logical deductions from their findings.

(viii) Indicated where appropriate either in the patient's history or in discussion the need for further investigative techniques.

(ix)   Demonstrated in their final determination of each case a logical response to the patient's history and symptoms and their ability to take into account a practitioner's legal and professional responsibilities.

(x)   Advised the patient about the use of the correction and recorded advice.'

Comments

Essentially, during the Routine PQE the examiners are looking for fitness to practise. To achieve this you need to perform a smooth, logical, safe routine eye examination. It is worth pointing out that there are two main areas that if performed poorly result in instant failure of this section:

1 Ophthalmoscopy: you will fail if this is deemed to be UNSAFE, i.e. you either miss an abnormality or perform the technique of ophthalmoscopy in such a way as to be likely to miss an abnormality.
2 Visual status of patient: in other words, you need to find accurately the refractive error and visual acuity. If the acuity is below normal standards (in most circumstances less than 6/9) you need to have a reason or suspicion as to the cause of the reduced acuity. This suspicion of cause of reduced acuity will give you a clue as to your management. For example: (a) reduced acuity due to cataract – perhaps refer for extraction; (b) reduced acuity due to longstanding strabismus – consider advice to patient on safety and inform GP; (c) reduced acuity due to pathology – refer appropriately.

13.2 THE EXAMINATION FORMAT

In most circumstances you will be in a centre that you may not have visited before. Therefore if you have any opportunity to visit the clinical areas of the test centres at the universities or at the Institute of Optometry before the exams, this will serve to orientate you and help in your preparation.

Each centre will have been sent a list of equipment that needs to be supplied for the routine exam. This includes:

• Test chart (note fan and block charts may not be present)
• Trial case with prisms, pinhole, Maddox rod and occluder
• RAF rule
• Near reading chart
• Halberg clips
• Maddox wing
• Mallett units

You need to take the following:

• Ophthalmoscope and retinoscope (charged or with spare batteries and bulbs)
• Trial frame
• Occluder and near fixation target, e.g. reduced Snellen letters
• Click-on click-off pen torch
• Crossed cyls
• Twirls

- Confirmation lenses
- Confrontation target
- Measuring tape
- PD/frame rule

The centre may supply a phoropter if you prefer, but ensure in advance of the exam that this can be arranged by the CO examinations co-ordinator.

You will have 45 minutes to examine a pre-presbyopic patient and 45 minutes to examine a presbyopic patient. Due to the arrangement of the exam you do not know which you will examine first. One examiner will supervise you for one patient and then you will have another examiner for the other patient. The examiners will pass on information to each other regarding your performance on the first patient, e.g. 'Watch his ophthalmoscopy/retinoscopy technique or check her cover test'. This means that although you may do poorly for the first patient you have a chance to shine in your performance on the second! However, the examiners will not tell you where you have gone wrong with the first patient.

Familiarize yourself with the routine exam sheet that will be sent to you by the CO at the beginning of your pre-registration year. Remember that you can regard this as a 'blank' sheet and insert your own labels and headings, with the proviso that these need to be clear and legible. Often this is the best approach because you will not be used to working from the CO record sheet.

13.3 WHAT DO THE EXAMINERS SAY?

(a) What advice would you give to a candidate preparing for the exam?
- Have several mock exams
  Many examiners have commented that candidates seem not to have had a mock exam. Arrange this with your supervisor and any other supervisors and optometrists you can so that your routine can be thoroughly assessed and 'dissected'. Ensure this is done several times and well in advance of the examination, so you have an opportunity to change or improve your performance.
- Practise explaining and justifying your test and results
  Keep asking yourself, 'why am I doing this test, is it objective, subjective, what do the results mean?' Compare the symptoms and history with your procedures. For example, the patient reports sore itchy eyes – do slit lamp exam with fluorescein (or in the exam suggest doing it!); the patient has family history of glaucoma therefore suggest fields and tonometry.
- Practise the timing of your routine
  In general you will take around 90 minutes to perform an eye examination at the start of your training year, while ten weeks into your pre-registration year you may take around an hour. Try to get

down to 35 or 40 minutes by the January or February before the exams to ensure you have spare time if things go wrong on the day of the PQE. Remember you can ask the examiner to give you a time check during the exam, but it is best to take a watch or a clock. Also, remember to do ophthalmoscopy early in the exam rather than at the end; you will fail instantly if you do not have enough time to do ophthalmoscopy.

- Bring along all equipment needed to examine the patient
  Nothing will upset an examiner more than a candidate arriving to see a patient without a retinoscope, trial frame or occluder for cover testing. Bring more than you need rather than less and ALWAYS have spare batteries, handles or bulbs.
- Have mocks in unfamiliar places
  Try to work in a different room, and from right and left sides of your patients if you can. This may only be possible for some trainees by doing volunteer work at another establishment, i.e. another practice, hospital or the Institute of Optometry. Remember you may be in an unfamiliar cubicle in the exam and it can be helpful to get used to the feeling of working somewhere different.
- Don't insert new parts into the routine
  It will take approximately two weeks for most pre-registration candidates to become accustomed to a new procedure inserted into the routine. Your exam routine procedures should appear 'smooth' and logical.
  Remember you must be 'fit to practise'. Although it would be excellent to be perfect, you don't have to be. But you do have to be safe. Keep this in mind when examining your patient and especially when deciding on management. Ask yourself 'have I done everything I need to and is my management and advice safe?'

(b) What areas of the subject require:
  (i) Sound knowledge?
    - Ophthalmoscopy
    - Symptoms and history
    - Referral criteria
    - Legal responsibilities
    - Recognition of ocular and systemic disease, especially if sight threatening
  (ii) and (iii) Reasonable knowledge and some knowledge?
    Not really appropriate to the routine PQE. This exam is intended for assessment of your day-to-day performance in eye examinations. You should perform well and demonstrate adequate knowledge in all areas of general examination sufficient to safely examine and manage patients.

(c) Successful candidates will have:
- Competence, common sense and confidence
- Good communication skills
- Sound knowledge of what they are doing and why
- Logical and fluent order of tests and procedures
- Safety.

(d) Candidates' marks are brought down by:
- Sarcasm, silence, stupidity
- Reticence in answering questions
- Illogical order or methods of tests
- Poor techniques
- Running out of time or spending too much time on one test
- Poor record keeping.

(e) Common causes of failure:
- Being unsafe to practise, e.g. poor ophthalmoscopic technique, missing ocular abnormalities or strabismus
- Failure to refer when appropriate and poor timing of referrals
- Poor, inadequate or absent management of the patient
- Not completing the assessment
- Poor record keeping.

13.4 HELP AND ADVICE

Preparing for the routine PQE starts as soon as your pre-registration year starts and concludes just before you enter the exam room.

At the start of your pre-registration year, ensure you are watched, checked and questioned on every patient until you feel happy to be left for longer periods on your own. Remember you should (hopefully!) only have one pre-registration year in your career. It is literally a unique experience. It is up to you personally to ensure you get the best out of this year. Tip: your supervisor should set out rules and regulations for you but also set yourself rules and a study plan and ask for more help, mock exams and homework.

Throughout your pre-registration year revise a different subject each week, e.g. binocular balancing, near adds, prescription analysis, and get into the habit of reading around the subject and studying straight away. This means that when you start to revise you really are doing just that and not learning from scratch a weekend before the exam. Tip: read the *Optician*, *OT* and other journals regularly. Also, when you see a patient with, say, glaucoma, revise glaucoma the same day. This reinforces your learning because you will relate what you learn to actual patients. Talk to pre-registration colleagues and other supervisors about interesting or difficult cases.

Ask several qualified optometrists what their management would be; every examiner is different. Ask questions all the time; you have a BSc after your name, therefore behave like a scientist and ask why, what and when from your colleagues.

Two months before your routine PQE, ensure your equipment is functioning and you have spare retinoscope and ophthalmoscope bulbs. If not, you have enough time to order and receive them. Nothing is more stressful than a PQE exam, except a PQE exam where your equipment or instruments fail. In the month before your exam you will probably not have had anyone sit in for a while on your routine. It is vital that you get someone not only to watch but also to criticize and advise you for several patients. Also try to work in an unfamiliar room or cubicle. Remember your examination room may not be familiar territory. Tip: have as many mock exams as you can arrange.

The night before the routine exam: do your last minute cramming! Double and triple check your exam equipment, i.e. your clothes, conservative, professional and clean; your instruments, working and with spare batteries and bulbs. Go to bed at a reasonable time; staying up late to revise will worry you, tire you and increase the risk of sleeping in.

On the morning of the exam, leave plenty of time to get to the venue. Eat or drink something that will give you energy.

Just before going in to the exam take three deep breaths. Good luck!

Model routine

The following is a concise 'model routine', which lists the basic procedures that should be carried out (if appropriate) and the considerations that the examiners will have. It is not meant to be exhaustive or prescriptive.

History and symptoms

It is often stated that 70 per cent of diagnoses can be made after a full and complete history and symptoms. The examiners will check that you ask relevant questions, follow up answers with subsequent questions and obtain sufficient information about any areas of interest that arise. Establish the reason for the visit (patients are primed to say they have lost their glasses), what were the glasses used for, any ocular symptoms, how is the distance and near vision with and without spectacles. Any allergies, headaches, diplopia, flashes or floaters or physical signs. Ocular history, spectacles, strabismus, eye disease or injury. General health, diabetes, blood pressure and such like. Medication, family history, ocular and general health. Occupation, hobbies, sports, driver, VDU user? Look for lid and pupil abnormalities as well as compensatory head postures when conducting your history and symptoms.

Examination of eyes and visual system

The examiners will look for a smooth and logical sequence of tests that should only be performed if appropriate. The candidate should appear adept at performing adequate examination techniques and obtain accurate results.

- Unaided visions, right, left and both eyes together
- Cover test distance and near
- Motility
- Pupil reactions
- NPC and accommodative amplitude if appropriate (for some patients these tests are best done after the subjective refraction with the new prescription in place)
- Assessment of peripheral fields using white 5 mm or red 15 mm target at 33 cm, confrontation or peripheral fields but not a combination of both, and know the extent of the normal monocular visual field
- Anterior segment examination using direct ophthalmoscope with broad beam. Exterior eye, lids, lashes, conjunctiva, cornea, iris, ask patient to look in primary position of gaze and then along four main meridians. During ophthalmoscopy, get very close to the patient's eye, lift upper lid when patient is looking down (warn patient before doing this), and examine the inferior media and fundus in nine positions of gaze. Observe the optic nerve head, colour, cup-to-disc ratio, neuro-retinal rim colour and form, and the disc margins; then the background and finally the macula.

Refraction

Again the examiners will look for a logical sequence of appropriate and properly performed techniques, leading to accurate results.

- Measure pupillary distance, set trial frame. Is the patient looking through the middle of the trial frame?
- Retinoscopy, use appropriate working distance and work on axis
- Subjective refraction (binocular when appropriate, e.g. young hyperope)
- Distance VA, binocular balancing
- Distance ocular motility balance (OMB), cover test or Maddox rod
- Mallett unit
- Near tests, working distance for patient's near tasks, amplitudes of accommodation, add(s), near balance, near VA, range of clear near vision, intermediate vision?
- Near OMB and binocular function, cover test or Maddox wing, Mallett, and stereo-tests?
- Supplementary tests should be performed if time and equipment allow, or written in the 'supplementary tests advised' box on the examination record sheet. Tonometry, field examination, slit lamp examination (with fluorescein and rose Bengal), colour vision, Amsler charts, cycloplegia, mydriasis
- Write down the final prescription.

Management

The examiners will look to see that you have assessed the patient's problems, presented the correct management options in a logical sequence, and clearly and concisely explained the situation to the patient. It should be established that the patient has understood your explanations and they should be given the opportunity to ask questions and discuss management options. Be clear and concise, avoid being repetitive or redundant, and do not offer conclusions that are not backed up by the data available. Treat the patient with courtesy and respect. Write the prescription with comments on suggested types of lenses, centration details, and instructions for use. Refer to or inform the GP if necessary. Give a prescription or statement to the patient or say that you would do so in your everyday practice. Advise as to the timing of the next eye examination. Make sure you have given all necessary advice to the patient verbally and written it all down.

13.5 PAST EXAM QUESTIONS

After you have completed eye examinations on both patients, the examiners will ask you questions about your technique or the patients you have just seen. Almost any question could come up during this part of the routine PQE, depending on the patients. Remember to 'dispose' of the patients properly, following this format:

1 Verbal advice and explanation to the patient
2 Written advice and explanation to patient
3 Issue a prescription and statement or say that you would
4 Suggest further tests, such as visual fields, tonometry, slit lamp and fluorescein, colour vision, Amsler charts, mydriatic and fundoscopy with slit lamp or binocular indirect ophthalmoscopy, cycloplegic refraction and such like.

The following is a short list of questions that have been asked in the past:

1 What would you do if you couldn't test pupil reactions with a pen torch, e.g. dark iridies?
2 Why is the testing of pupils important?
3 If someone had a red eye and had recently been abroad, what could this mean and what could you do about it?
4 Specific questions about presbyopia
5 Would you be happy dispensing the obtained refraction?
6 How do you do binocular balancing?
7 If the patient is using a multi-pinhole, would the refraction be affected if they are looking through two holes at once?
8 What else would you have done? (If you ran out of time)

9 How did you assess the stability of fusion? Did you look at the recovery after cover test?

10 How does nystagmus affect vision? How would you modify your routine when assessing a patient with nystagmus?

Common queries from candidates regarding the routine exam:

1 Do I record vision?
   Yes, the patient will have their correction removed and so this will be a legal requirement. It also gives a clue to the patient's refractive error, e.g. 6/18 and N5 is suggestive of −1.00 D myopia.

2 If vision is poor do I do cover test?
   Yes, but remember to mention to the examiner the limitations of your test, e.g. 'I know it wasn't an accommodative target but I felt that the information would be useful'. Use a spotlight target when the distance visual acuity is equal to or less than 6/18.

3 Do I have correction in place to do confrontation or assessment of peripheral fields?
   No, the patient will have been told to say that they've lost or broken their glasses and you cannot do these tests with trial lenses!

4 What do I use to examine the external eye?
   You can use several procedures here. Slit lamp, if this is available and you can competently complete the external examination in time. This is probably the best method (just asking or mentioning you would like to use a slit lamp may give you extra credibility). Ophthalmoscope, use a wide beam and ask the patient to look up, down, right and left. Remember to lift the lid on down-gaze. It is probably best to have a good look at the external eye while doing ophthalmoscopy and suggest slit lamp examination.

5 What do I use for a confrontation target?
   Use a target that simulates the standard target for the Goldmann or Humphrey field analyser, i.e. Goldmann III target 5 mm diameter. A white spot target on a black thin stick would be acceptable. Remember to mention the limitations of the test, i.e. 'It is a gross test and a field test performed on a perimeter would be preferable'.

6 What do I use for motility?
   A pen torch; you can observe corneal reflexes. Remember to incorporate the cover test and to test for ductions when a mechanical restriction is suspected.

7 Shall I do ophthalmoscopy at the end?
   I would advise against this for two reasons. First the ophthalmoscopic appearance may help to explain refractive findings. Second if you run out of time and fail to finish ophthalmoscopy then you fail, full stop.

8 If my presbyope is 60 years old, should I measure accommodation?
   No, the patient will have no clinically usable accommodation, so it would

be more logical to 'guesstimate' the first lens to determine the add and then check the range of clear near vision that this provides.

9 Can I put a tick or 'NAD' if everything appears normal?
No, a tick means that the tissue you are looking at 'existed' but does not describe its appearance. As for NAD, most examiners feel that this translates as 'Not Actually Done'! Record appearances as 'normal' or write a brief description, e.g. cornea – clear, bright reflex.

10 Do I measure NPC on a presbyopic patient?
Yes, but if they are uncorrected (which is the case in the routine PQE) and are hyperopic you need to advise the patient that the target may be blurred. If the near visions are such that the patient cannot see your NPC target, do the test with the near refraction in place (adjust the trial frame so that the patient can still see the target with both eyes as it approaches).

13.6 MORE INFO?

Elliott, D. *Clinical Procedures in Primary Eye Care*, second edition. Oxford: Butterworth-Heinemann, 2003.

Edwards, K and Llewllyn, R. *Optometry*. Oxford: Butterworth, 1988.

Case records and law

Nu Nu Braddick

14.1 WHAT DOES THE CO SAY?

The following information is taken from the CO pre-registration pack. The syllabus is short and to the point: 'An examination based on case records submitted by a candidate, which will also include discussion of the practitioner's responsibility under current legislation.'

The GOC do not provide a specific core curriculum/core competencies for case studies and law examination but some information on standards can be found in the curriculum for Core Subject 2: Professional Conduct (find it in your pre-registration pack supplied by the CO). This will help you determine the standard you need to achieve in this subject.

The CO provide information under three headings: fitness to practise, nature of the examination and assessment.

Fitness to practice

'Success in the Case Records and Law section must indicate that the candidate possesses:

(i)   An understanding of the importance of adequate and accurate records sufficient to demonstrate competence in patient management.
(ii) A breadth of experience obtained since graduation, which extends over the whole field of optometry.
(iii) A knowledge of the regulation of the Optometric profession and an understanding of general law adequate to enable safe, legal practice.'

Nature of the examination

'There will be an oral examination for 30 minutes with two examiners. Each candidate should submit 20 case records. Of the 20 records submitted, 10 MUST represent one each chosen from the 21 categories listed below and be annotated accordingly. The remaining 10 may be included at the candidate's discretion to demonstrate the full extent of their experience during the pre-registration year. Figures in brackets are for guidance only.

1 Child (under 8 years)
2 Cycloplegic refraction
3 High myopia (greater than 8 D)
4 High hypermetropia/aphakia (greater than 8 D)
5 Protective spectacles dispensed
6 Use of mydriatic
7 LVA/magnifier dispensed
8 Referral of abnormal ocular condition
9 Visual fields assessment
10 Contact lenses
11 Occupation specific prescribing (e.g. VDU)
12 Colour vision anomaly
13 Anisometropia (greater than 2 D)
14 Heterotropia
15 Uncompensated heterophoria
16 Ocular emergency
17 Non-tolerance to prescription
18 Management of the elderly patient
19 Detection of systemic disease
20 Investigation of suspect glaucoma
21 Pseudophakia
22 ADDRS card submitted.'

Assessment

'In every case the examiners will look to see that the candidate has demonstrated:

(i)   Full and complete records that show a sound and consistent basic examination technique (and can justify the fullness or otherwise of each record).

(ii) An awareness of the need for flexibility of approach with the use of supplementary examinations where indicated.

(iii) That the full implications of symptoms and history, and examination results have been appreciated and acted upon, with the possibility of alternative approaches to management considered.

(iv) From the records, that the legal and professional responsibilities have been met.

(v)   (a) A knowledge of all legal obligations, including the Opticians Act, GOC rules and principles, the GOS regulations (bearing in mind regional variations) and the law directly relevant to the practice of optometry in the United Kingdom (even though it may

be the candidate's intention never to practise in the United Kingdom).
(b) A broad understanding of Contract Law, the Law of Negligence, and Consumer Protection Legislation.
(c) A knowledge of the existence of employment and business legislation, Shops and Offices Acts, Insurance requirements, etc. and how this legislation may be relevant to the practice of optometry.

14.2 THE EXAMINATION FORMAT

Case Records and Law is probably the only PQE in which the candidate is able to select topics (i.e. the case records) to be discussed during the examination and therefore have a good idea of the questions that are likely to be asked. The examiners will have the case records that were submitted by you earlier in the year. You should have a copy of your own to refer to during the examination. A template for the case records format can be found on the CD-ROM sent to you by the CO or downloaded from the CO website. Points of discussion will largely depend on the type of cases submitted. See Section 14.4 Help and Advice below for advice on case selection and preparation of case records.

Most of the 30-minute examination will be spent discussing points raised from the records and questions on law tend to take up the last few minutes of this examination. However, the law questions are not to be underestimated and must be answered competently to pass the examination!

14.3 WHAT DO THE EXAMINERS SAY?

Several examiners were asked to comment on the case records and law PQE and the following is an assimilation of their responses.

(a) What advice would you give to a candidate preparing for the exam?
All examiners stressed the need to read the CO guidelines and syllabus thoroughly. Many also suggested asking other optometrists, other than your supervisor, to read through the records in order to obtain several opinions on the presentation of your cases. Ask for a mock viva on a few case records. It is recommended that you start collecting potential case studies at the beginning of the pre-registration year. One examiner suggested aiming to complete all records by the end of January!
(b) What areas of the subject require:
(i) Sound knowledge?
Candidates should be fully aware of all the legal and professional obligations in practice. Sound knowledge of professional bodies and their functions is essential, including an understanding of the difference between GOC and local legislation.

(ii) Reasonable knowledge?
Candidates should cover the subjects of professional indemnity and insurance, the Health and Safety Act, Shops and Railway Premises Act, laws relating to negligence, data protection, VAT, consumer law, employment law.

(iii) Some knowledge?
A basic knowledge of laws of contract and disciplinary procedures is required.

(c) What do you look for in the successful candidate?
Examiners look for competent individuals who show good reasoning ability and are confident in their explanations of all the tests carried out and of the findings recorded. Neat and well-presented (but not necessarily typed) records will pre-dispose most examiners favourably. On individual case questions, candidates must be able to answer with convincing recollection of REAL patients and provide appropriate supporting comments. Overall, the case records and viva should reveal a year of good all-round optometric experience.

(d) What brings marks down?
Examiners will not look favourably on poorly presented records, silly mistakes such as vision that does not correlate with the prescription, and absence of appropriate detail, e.g. date of current prescription or dosage of medication. The candidate will also lose marks if a logical explanation cannot be provided for unusual results in certain tests. The candidate should be confident in the selection of particular methods of testing and will again lose marks if he/she does not appear to know why such tests are carried out. Examiners will not be impressed with over-confidence, especially if this means potentially unsafe practice! Slow and vague replies in the viva will find the examiners impatient. You should perhaps 'think out loud' if there is a delay in replying with the required answer. Generally, marks can be lost for any indication that the candidate is ill-prepared.

(e) What are the common causes of failure?
Examiners will fail candidates lacking in awareness of professional responsibilities that would indicate potentially unsafe practice, e.g. if the candidate noted an unusual finding but failed to investigate further or refer.

(f) What subjects do candidates place too little importance upon?
Examiners feel that candidates are generally too dismissive of non-optometric law and law in direct relation to practice and patients. Candidates should also be more aware of follow-up procedures for referred patients. The record of patients' history and symptoms should be sufficiently detailed, e.g. if the patient is on medication the duration and dosage taken must be noted, frequency and severity of

symptoms must be noted, and full specification of the patient's existing spectacle prescription, including optical centres and VA, must also be noted.

(g) Any other comments?

Early in the pre-registration year the candidate should organize a revision plan and discuss topics with the supervisor, other optometrists and fellow pre-registration optometrists. It is also suggested that a greater number of case records than necessary should be collected in order to improve the variety of the cases and eventually to select the best 20. One suggestion is to complete five cases in December, five in January, five in February and five in March. Neat and sensible dress is recommended even though no patients will be encountered.

14.4 HELP AND ADVICE

Case records

Candidates should begin collecting potential case records early on in the pre-registration year. The final 20 cases chosen should eventually cover more than ten of the categories listed by the CO, for you will probably have examined patients from most if not all of the categories. It is important to remember that the type of cases submitted should be reflective of your experience throughout the year. Therefore examiners do not expect to find weird and wonderful cases in the records! It is recommended you keep a selection of typical 'everyday' cases, such as investigation of glaucoma, visual field assessments, binocular vision problems, and VDU eye examinations.

In each category, it is not advisable to be too adventurous, e.g. in contact lens cases it is probably best to avoid controversial topics such as monovision or extended wear. Perhaps a typical case, one each of a gas permeable and a soft lens fitting, would be adequate. Remember that the questions in the viva will be based on the particular cases submitted and the more complex the cases, the more in-depth the questions are likely to be. Do not be too ambitious! However, it is important that the candidate should not avoid cases that involve important aspects of optometric practice, such as diabetic patients, glaucoma, referrals (emergency and non-urgent) and such like. Examiners will be very concerned if, of the 20 records submitted, none of the cases dealt with any of these aspects.

As stated above, all records should be adequately detailed. If necessary, contact the patient after the eye examination, to confirm the information given for history and symptoms. The following is a 'checklist' to help prevent commonly made errors:

1 Unaided vision must correlate with refractive results.
2 Drug name, dosage and duration of any medication must be recorded.

3 Where appropriate, dates of any previous ocular treatment should be recorded.
4 Frequency, severity and duration of symptoms must be noted.
5 Patient's current prescription must be fully recorded, including date prescribed, optical centres, type of lens, VA achieved, etc.
6 Ophthalmoscopic findings, pathological or otherwise, should be recorded in full detail, i.e. positive information should not be noted as NAD (nothing abnormal detected)! Any unusual features of the fundus should be specifically noted according to size (as a ratio of disc diameter), colour, depth, and location.
7 For prescriptions of 5 DS or above the back vertex distance should be specified.
8 Where appropriate, intra-ocular pressure readings should be specified by time and type of tonometer, and note the anaesthetic used for applanation tonometry.
9 Copies of referral letters should not reveal any of the patient's personal details e.g. full name, address, GP. Such information should be deleted from all photocopies of letters submitted with the records.
10 In contact lens cases, full specification of all lenses involved should be recorded, such as the lens make and design, lens material and lens parameters, and any tints or coatings. All lens solutions involved should also be noted in the record. If fluorescein is instilled then record it!
11 Where applicable, keratometry readings should correspond to the prescription and fitting combination.
12 Remember always to include the main reason that the patient has presented for an eye examination. If this was because of a visual problem, then this must be addressed in the management plan.

The records must be submitted as two sets of ten (usually with one contact lens case in each set) and must be numbered 1 to 20. Each set should contain a reasonable range of topics. A summary sheet of all 20 case records should accompany each set. It is strongly advised that each set of case records should also be accompanied by a key to the abbreviations used in the records. Candidates should try to complete the case records by March. If you aim to complete them EARLY, you are more likely to complete them ON TIME!

Law

Candidates should be fully aware of all legal and professional obligations in practice and must read and familiarize themselves with the role and specific functions of all governing bodies, including the GOC and the CO. Candidates should also be aware of the Opticians Act, GOS regulations including regional variation involving terms of service and ophthalmic lists, AOP guidelines especially those involving occupation-specific prescribing, e.g. VDU users.

Given the current changes in Europe, it is recommended that candidates should keep up to date with all aspects of law relevant to optometry. Candidates must also be familiar with the different categories of patients eligible for NHS eye examinations and the appropriate NHS forms involved, including the GOS(ST)A, GOS(P), GOS(V), GOS18, GOS2(R), and ST(V) forms.

14.5 PAST EXAM QUESTIONS

1 When is a letter to the GP necessary?
2 Which is more important, GOC rules or the Opticians Act?
3 What is the patient signing for on the GOS18 form?
4 Why do patients have to sign the GOS18 form? Is this a recent change?
5 Is it OK to use the GOS18 form for referring private patients?
6 What is the difference between a letter of information and a letter of referral?
7 If you examined someone who had an IOP on repeated testing of R 22 and L 24 mmHg, with normal optic discs and normal fields, what would your action be?
8 Which visual field screener do you use and how effective is it?
9 What would be your ideal visual field screener and why?
10 Why did/didn't you carry out a visual field assessment on a high myope?
11 A patient telephones to say that because he was kept longer than the agreed half hour for the eye test, he received a parking ticket and expects to be reimbursed for it or he will sue. Where do you stand legally? Is a contract binding when not written?
12 What does GOS stand for?
13 Which bodies do you need to register with in order to practice? Can you practice in the UK if you are not a member of the CO?
14 On passing your exams, what do you need to do before you can practise? Do you need professional indemnity cover and how would you arrange it?
15 What is the difference between GOC and local legislation?
16 What are the three reasons for which you can be removed from an ophthalmic list?
17 What is the OCCS?
18 Have you dispensed any eye protectors this year? What are your legal responsibilities?
19 What advice do you give to contact lens patients? Does this cover you if the patient suffers from a corneal ulcer and loses vision in one eye?
20 If a patient persisted in driving despite your advising him/her that their vision is inadequate, would you inform the DVLA, or police, or anybody?
21 You receive a letter from a solicitor whose client is considering taking legal action against you. The solicitor requires a copy of the patient's records. What do you do?

22 A patient walks into your practice demanding his/her case records. What do you do?

23 What laws other than the Opticians Act must opticians comply with in everyday practice?

24 What is a contract?

25 What could you do if somebody refused to pay for their sight test or refused to collect their glasses? What would you do?

26 How would your legal obligations differ when performing an NHS sight test as opposed to a private sight test?

27 You examine an elderly patient and find their vision to be satisfactory and the patient is happy. The eyes are healthy but you note early lenticular opacities. Would you;
   (a) Inform the patient?
   (b) Inform the GP?
   (c) See again in 12 months?
   (d) All three?

28 A patient walks into your practice with a receipt for payment for a pair of glasses bought two years ago. The patient is asking for reimbursement because the lenses are scratched. What would you do?

29 Do patients have to pay VAT on spectacles now?

30 If you refer a patient for cataracts and the ophthalmologist additionally diagnoses glaucoma, how do you stand legally?

31 How would you stand if the ophthalmologist found that you had missed:
   (a) Anterior uveitis?
   (b) Retinal tear?

32 What is the legal position of an optometrist who recommends nutritional supplements?

33 Can an optometrist prescribe all types of POM?

34 What is a signed order?

35 Which professional takes the responsibility for a signed order supplied on a POM?

36 What do you understand by the term shared-care?

37 Do you have to be registered with the CO in order to practise?

38 Do you have to be registered with the GOC in order to practise?

39 Do you have to be a member of the AOP in order to practise?

40 What is meant by the term indemnity insurance?

41 What is a good source of information on employment law?

42 If a company agrees over the phone to provide you with locum work for one day but cancel on the day you arrive in practice, has a contract been broken?

43 If you fail to turn up for a locum day that has been agreed over the phone, has a contract been broken?

44 Is VAT payable on an eye examination fee?

45 What is meant by post-payment verification?

46 If a person falls on some stairs in your practice, despite there being a sign advising 'take care', are you obliged to pay compensation?

47 Are there any employment laws that restrict the opening times of optometry practices?

48 What is the difference between the titles optometrist and optician?

49 Can a GP issue a prescription for glasses?

50 Can an ophthalmologist issue a prescription for contact lenses?

51 A patient that you advised to have LASIK undergoes the procedure but is not happy with the outcome. Are you obliged to pay them compensation?

52 A refractive surgeon offers to provide you with a 'finders fee' for each patient you refer for refractive surgery. Is this legal?

53 Can an unqualified person supply glasses to a person who is registered partially sighted?

54 Can an unqualified person supply glasses to anyone?

55 Under what circumstances can a dispensing optician supply contact lenses?

56 Can a dispensing optician supply low vision devices?

57 Under what circumstances could you re-examine a child after one month and claim an NHS fee?

58 Can a spectacle voucher be supplied for plano tinted spectacle lenses?

59 Are plano coloured contact lenses classed as a medical device?

60 Is it legal for non-ophthalmic outlets to sell plano coloured contact lenses?

61 Is it legal to prescribe R and L $+0.25/-0.25 \times 75$?

Questions on case records can be very diverse. Any mistakes or inconsistencies will be queried. If you see that you have made a mistake then admit it. Perhaps say that with the benefit of further experience you would modify your actions in future.

It is a good idea to know the areas that your case records cover, e.g. diabetes/ use of drugs, because the examiners will probably ask questions about these topics.

14.6 MORE INFO?

Taylor, S. *Law in Optometric Practice*. Oxford: Butterworth-Heinemann, 2002.

College of Optometrists. *Code of Ethics and Guidelines for Professional Conduct*. College of Optometrists, 1991.

The Opticians Act. HMSO, 1989.

15

Ocular disease and abnormality

Simon Brooks

15.1 WHAT DOES THE CO SAY?

The following information is taken from the CO pre-registration pack. The information in italics is my own and not provided by the CO. The syllabus is short and to the point: 'The recognition and differentiation of abnormal conditions of the eyes, adnexa, and visual system and ocular signs of systemic disorders. The recognition of cases to be referred for medical opinion and the relative urgency of referral. The normal appearance of the structure of the eye and adnexa with physiological variations and the ageing eye.'

The GOC do provide specific core curriculum/core competencies for ocular disease and abnormality and information on standards can be found in the curriculum for Core Subject 6: Ocular Abnormalities (find it in your pre-registration pack supplied by the CO). This will help you determine the standard you need to achieve in this subject.

The CO provide information under three headings: fitness to practise, nature of the examination and assessment.

Fitness to practise

'In optometric practice practitioners must be able to detect abnormal ocular conditions (at an early as well as late stage in their course) and to differentiate the abnormal from the normal eye. They must be able to recognize the need for referral or reporting, to judge the relative urgency thereof, and to be familiar in every case with the appropriate method of referral or reporting.'

Nature of the examination

'The examination will be in two parts.

(i) Practical
     This exam is in the form of a modified station examination. Candidates
     will be asked to complete eight tasks, which might include the

examination of patients. These tasks may include examination of patients, assessment of slides and consideration of the results of a variety of patient investigations. Five minutes will be allotted to each task.

(ii) Oral

This part of the exam lasts 20 minutes and will be with two examiners. Where the oral exam follows the practical it may commence with the candidate being asked to discuss the results of the tasks performed during the station examination. This will then extend to a more general discussion.'

Assessment

'In every case the examiners will look to see that candidates have:

(i)   Demonstrated accurate observation.
(ii)   Not failed to recognize any significant sign or symptom.
(iii) Made logical deductions from their findings.
(iv)   Related visual defects to ocular pathology with an ability to suggest a possible prognosis with particular reference to the incidence of ocular diseases.
(v)   Searched for possible secondary to primary conditions (e.g. glaucoma following uveitis).
(vi)   Related ocular findings to possible systemic disease.
(vii) Indicated (where appropriate) the need for and urgency of referral or reporting and a familiarity with the procedures thereof.'

15.2 THE EXAMINATION FORMAT

The examination is split into two parts, and either practical or oral may come first. During the practical exam there will be an invigilator (known as the 'ring master'), much the same as the Dispensing practical (which is also a station exam). At each station there will be a brief outline of the history of the case (and it will be brief – one or two lines perhaps – be careful, for most relevant information may not be immediately obvious). You will be required to describe what you see, to give your diagnosis and the management you propose. Here you can't be too cautious – all cases are likely to have some abnormality, and even if it is not pathological should still require a letter informing the patient's GP.

The five-minute period must allow enough time to read through the brief history and either examine the image, or if the task involves the examination of a patient, slit lamp biomicroscopy or ophthalmoscopy – still leaving enough time to write your findings down. Work swiftly through the exam and do not be too concerned if you cannot arrive at a firm diagnosis. For this exam the most important thing is to recognize that something is abnormal and to know how it should be investigated and managed. Familiarize yourself with the record sheet to be used in the exam, which should have been sent to you by the CO. This has three boxes for you to write in:

1 Please describe what you have seen.
2 Based on the case history given and your observations above, indicate your provisional diagnosis.
3 Indicate your immediate management of the patient.

The 20 -minute oral examination may begin with a discussion of one or more cases encountered in the practical if this part is taken subsequently, although in my experience this rarely happens. However, this is a broad subject and therefore examiners will try to work through as many aspects as possible. Common sight-threatening and treatable eye diseases tend to require greater depth of knowledge than unusual conditions or rare syndromes. Questions may vary from asking about differential diagnosis of certain abnormalities to surgical techniques and possible complications.

15.3 WHAT DO THE EXAMINERS SAY?

The following comments are assimilated from the responses of several examiners.

(a) What advice would you give to a candidate preparing for the exam?
It is important for the candidate to understand the significance of what they see in the eye. They must revise basic anatomy and physiology and relate it to disease aetiology. It is also necessary to classify referrals – routine, urgent and emergency. Study sight- or life-threatening conditions thoroughly as these are pass or fail areas. Think about how a disease may present in the practice. Discuss cases with your supervisor and fellow students and if possible with an ophthalmologist.

(b) What areas of the subject require:
(i)   Sound knowledge?
Aetiology, signs, symptoms and referral criteria for common treatable sight-threatening (or life-threatening) diseases, e.g. glaucoma, diabetic eye disease, cataract, and also methods of examination – when to dilate, assess fields and so on, and knowledge of management of certain conditions that the optometrist might be asked to monitor after informing the GP, e.g. ocular hypertension.

(ii) Reasonable knowledge?
Pharmacological and surgical treatment of all eye diseases, but especially the more common occurrences. Surgical techniques and complications, especially cataract operations. Systemic medication and ocular side effects. Pupil defects and neurology.

(iii) Some knowledge?
Diseases not often encountered, especially those that eventually become so obvious that they will be diagnosed but where early or late diagnosis does not affect prognosis. Many hereditary disorders fit this description. Supplementary methods of examination used by the ophthalmologist, especially fundus photography and fluorescein angiography.

(c) What do you look for in the successful candidate?
Practical management of every-day situations and confidence with management; if a candidate doesn't know, then they show they are prepared to refer to text books or seek advice from the GP or ophthalmologist.

(d) What brings people's marks down?
Confident statements that are wrong, and throwaway statements that cannot be backed up, such as 'I would dilate all patients even if it wasn't clinically justified just for my own practice'. Dangerous management. Prevarication by candidates who are aware that they are lacking and try to highjack (*sic*) the exams by dramatics and other delaying tactics.

One examiner states that 'bigheaded overconfidence and sarcastic remarks to the examiner which rubs (*sic*) him up the wrong way' as a reason for bringing marks down. I find it difficult to believe that anybody in the situation that a PQE candidate is in when taking the exams would be sarcastic to the examiner. However, this demonstrates the importance of thinking carefully about your answers and communicating them in a logical and professional manner so that they cannot be misconstrued.

(e) What are the commonest causes of failure?
Lack of basic knowledge or a disorganized, unprofessional attitude. In our opinion, a very important point was raised by one examiner, namely, the inability to perceive a serious condition in a common symptom and thus not take management seriously. Not referring a possible medical emergency appropriately is an instant failure. However, it is unlikely that you would be failed for not knowing about rare diseases.

(f) What subject areas do candidates place too little importance on?
Related anatomy and physiology, and how the aetiology of a disease affects prognosis and referral criteria. How pathology would present in practice.

(g) Any other comments?
Students should not expect to be examined in every detail on obscure ocular diseases. Rather they should leave the examiner with the overall impression that basic fundamentals of aetiology, recognition of signs and symptoms, and principles of management are well understood. The candidate should ensure that more common life- or sight-threatening

conditions, where early treatment is necessary for full recovery, are thoroughly understood. Note that because this is such a broad subject, rote learning doesn't work. The candidate should also understand that in practice presenting signs and symptoms might be very different from textbook cases.

15.4 HELP AND ADVICE

This is perhaps the only exam where students undertaking their pre-registration year in the HES are at a distinct advantage over those in private practice. However, those students in private practice should have at least one half-day session a week spent with an ophthalmologist in a clinic. Sometimes arrangements may be made for a block release of two weeks in a hospital, but I feel that continuous contact with an ophthalmologist throughout the whole year is more helpful – especially as it allows you to ask questions about cases you see each week in practice. However your time in the HES is arranged, it is important to spend this time wisely. Try to avoid being pushed into performing refractions while you are there. The purpose of the hospital experience is to gain as much knowledge as possible from the ophthalmologist, to gain an insight as to how her clinics are run, and what referral criteria are used in your area and what information is expected in referral letters and such like. If you are holding a hospital pre-registration position then it is likely that much of your time is spent refracting only, so make sure you are also allocated some premium time with an ophthalmologist.

During my pre-registration training I did not carry out a single refraction at the hospital. All of my time was spent with the ophthalmologist discussing each of his cases and usually he would ask questions. I found this approach extremely helpful in preparing for examiners questions.

The Practical

Equipment to take to the exam

Don't forget your ophthalmoscope and new batteries!

History

This brief outline may give a useful insight to the nature of the problem. However, be careful for it may equally be misleading – so don't jump to conclusions.

Examination of the image is fairly straightforward and will often be a textbook example of a particular abnormality; the image may even be straight out of one of Kanski's books. Watch for differential diagnoses and therefore different prognoses.

Examination of the patient

There is a possibility that in the pressurized atmosphere a candidate may make the simple blunder of examining the wrong eye, or less likely, the wrong segment. If you find an abnormality, don't assume it is the only abnormality. Do a thorough examination even if you spot something straight away, e.g. if you see an obvious fundus sign don't neglect to mention the presence of lenticular opacities.

Answering the questions

What do you see? Describe everything relevant, even if it is normal, e.g. if you have a background diabetic retinopathy with normal discs, describe the discs as well as the vasculature.

Diagnosis?

As I have said before, don't worry if you cannot give a firm diagnosis. If in your opinion there are two or three possible diagnoses then list the possibilities, and where appropriate suggest the tests you would carry out to differentiate between them.

Management?

This section is of course much easier if you have made a firm and accurate diagnosis, and accuracy is important. It is not enough to recognize diabetic retinopathy. You need to know how advanced the disease is in order to suggest an appropriate course of action. Probably your most likely management will be one of the following:

(i)   Inform the GP and patient and review in 3, 6 or 12 months
(ii) Refer to the GP
(iii) Refer to an ophthalmologist via the GP and in turn
(iv) Refer via the GP with a recommendation that the patient is seen soon
(v)   Refer direct to hospital and notify the GP of your action.

It is unlikely that any of the patients you see will require urgent referral (check history), but slides may of course include emergency conditions. Certainly there may be variations to these managements, e.g. the removal of a superficial foreign body might require a review the following day and a note to the GP, but may not require further follow up.

The oral

Attention to detail, especially in diabetic eye disease, glaucoma and cataract and also red eye, is very important. Be prepared for lateral thinking and working out from basic knowledge the answers to more obscure problems. Differential diagnosis and presentation in practice commonly cause the candidate problems. Don't mention obscure conditions unless you know them well, and if you do not know the answer to a question it is often worth admitting this. The examiner will usually change the topic or may guide you through working out the answer from facts that you do know. Of course if you are not sure what the examiner is asking then the same question may be rephrased more coherently. Often the question will be of the form where a patient attends with a particular symptom. While it is important not to dismiss common symptoms that may sometimes indicate very serious conditions, it is also important not to automatically assume the worst case scenario. A thirteen-year-old girl with bilateral visions of 6/18 but normal fundus signs is likely to be 1 dioptre myopic and unlikely to have a pituitary tumour. Remember the adage, 'if you hear hooves then it is probably horses because zebras are rare'. The examiner will lead from one topic to the next. Thinking out loud in a logical fashion usually gains encouragement from the examiner, and even if the candidate arrives at the wrong conclusion she will be encouraged to try again.

Be aware when preparing for this subject that there is some overlap with the Binocular Vision and Drugs exams.

Where to get experience

HES, specialist clinics – diabetic, orthoptic, laser and such like. In practice, write your own referral letters and learn to make your own decisions. You can do this by making a provisional decision and then checking with your supervisor. Confer on cases with fellow students at local optical society meetings and attend at least one refresher course geared to pre-registration students that dedicates a session to this exam.

One final point. Keep reading *OT* and *Optician*, for there will be a number of articles about ocular pathology throughout your year. Also it is important to keep up to date with the politics of the profession, for this may sometimes influence the topics examined, e.g. with the introduction of shared-care schemes for diabetic patients in many areas it has become even more important to assess the extent of retinopathy, and to know when the condition may be safely managed in the practice and when the condition must be referred.

15.5 PAST EXAM QUESTIONS

Most PQE questions are intended to provoke a conversation with the candidate. One-word answers are not expected; most examiners prefer a discussion and will prompt or guide the candidate where appropriate into greater depth or detail, or towards another subject.

1 Discuss different types of cataract, their causes and appearances.
2 What is the difference between wet and dry AMD?
3 What would you expect if you could see no red reflex on ophthalmoscopy? Name as many causes as possible.
4 A thirteen-year-old girl presents with bilateral reduced vision (6/18) but no fundus signs. What could be the problem?
5 A patient attends with a unilateral painful red eye present for the last five days. What could it be? How would you examine this patient?
6 How would you look for cells in the anterior chamber? What type of illumination would you use?
7 A patient has no vision in one eye and you notice that the other eye is developing disciform macular degeneration. Is disciform macular degeneration a disease that develops quickly? How would you manage this patient?
8 What is glaucoma?
9 Can iritis result in glaucoma? If so, is it of quick onset?
10 What sort of people are prone to glaucoma? Is this the same for chronic and acute?
11 A patient presents with floaters. What is your action and advice?
12 What conditions might warrant a direct referral?
13 How would you differentially diagnose acute ischaemic optic neuropathy and papilloedema?
14 What is a dystrophy? What corneal dystrophies do you know of?
15 What kinds of corneal ulceration are there? Are there any types associated with soft contact lens wear?
16 If a patient attends with a dendritic ulcer, why would you phone the GP, having already referred by letter?
17 How does diabetes affect blood vessels?
18 How would you examine a diabetic patient?
19 What fundus signs would indicate to you that the retinopathy is pre-proliferative, or proliferative?
20 What histologically are cotton wool spots?
21 What are the ocular features of thyroid eye disease?
22 A patient presents with unilateral sudden painless loss of vision. What are the possible causes? Describe the vascular supply to the eye.
23 How would you treat a red eye?
24 How would you look for a retinal detachment? What would you do on finding one?
25 What may cause inflammatory cells to be present in the vitreous?
26 How can the fundus be obscured?
27 Describe the phacoemulsification procedure. What other surgical techniques are used for cataract extractions and what are the possible complications? How may induced astigmatism be reduced?
28 What ocular conditions may contra-indicate cataract extraction surgery?

29 What are the symptoms of acute iritis and acute glaucoma?

30 What are micro-aneurysms? Can they be seen with an ophthalmoscope?

31 What do you know about the treatments for glaucoma?

32 How is proliferative diabetic retinopathy treated? What happens and how does it work?

33 What do you know about photorefractive keratotomy? What pathological condition is an Excimer laser sometimes used to treat?

34 A patient presents with a ptosis of one eyelid. How would you investigate this and what are the possible causes?

35 What diseases may affect the eyelids?

36 How might arthritis affect the eyes?

37 When would you refer a patient with cataract(s)?

38 How would you manage a patient with a family history of retinitis pigmentosa?

39 You examine a patient who is being treated with steroids. What are your considerations before performing contact tonometry or contact lens fitting?

40 A patient presents with a vesicular rash on one side of the face/head. What could it be? What indicates the likelihood of ocular involvement? How is the ocular condition treated?

41 What are the possible causes of dry eye syndrome? How may dry eye be treated?

42 What are the possible causes of sudden transient loss of vision? How would you differentiate?

43 How is nystagmus classified?

44 How might hypertension affect the eyes?

45 How would you manage the ocular hypertensive?

46 What are the main causes of ischaemic optic neuropathy? How is it treated?

47 A patient attends complaining of watery eyes but otherwise little discomfort. What are the possible causes and what would be your management?

48 How would you differentiate between scleritis and episcleritis? How does the management of these conditions differ?

49 A patient attends with a unilateral red eye. There appears to be no discomfort and vision seems unaffected. How would you manage this patient?

50 When is gonioscopy indicated?

51 What tumours may affect the eyelids?

52 What tumours may affect the fundus? Are they primary or secondary?

53 A patient returns having continuing problems with the reading glasses you have prescribed. You make all the appropriate checks (refraction, ocular motor balance, lens centration, etc.) and can find nothing wrong.

Furthermore, media and fundi appear normal. What additional tests would you carry out and what could the problem be?

54 Given the choice which would you prefer to have: herpes simplex or herpes zoster? What are the late complications of herpes zoster ophthalmicus?

55 What sort of people tend to have retinal detachments?

56 A patient attends with a sore watery eye but there is no redness. What is wrong with it?

57 What are soft exudates? In what sort of patient would you expect to see them?

58 What ocular problems are caused by diabetes?

59 What sort of vision would you expect in an amblyopic eye? How would you manage amblyopia?

60 What are the different causes of conjunctivitis? What do you know about antivirals?

15.6 MORE INFO?

Adams, G and Hubbard, A. *Kennerley Bankes's Clinical Ophthalmology: A Text and Colour Atlas*. Oxford: Butterworth-Heinemann, 1999.

Bruce, A, Loughnan, MS and Kanski, JJ. *Anterior Eye and Therapeutics A–Z*. Oxford: Butterworth-Heinemann, 2002.

Kanski, JJ. *Clinical Ophthalmology*. Fifth edition. Oxford: Butterworth-Heinemann, 2003.

Spalton, D. *Atlas of Clinical Ophthalmology*. Churchill-Livingstone, 1984.

Contact lenses

Mary Ware

16.1 WHAT DOES THE CO SAY?

The following information is taken from the CO pre-registration pack. The information in italics is my own and not provided by the CO. The syllabus is short and to the point: 'The prescribing and fitting of contact lenses and the management of contact lens patients.'

The GOC do provide specific core curriculum/core competencies for contact lenses and information on standards can be found in the curriculum or Core Subject 7: Contact Lenses (find it in your pre-registration pack supplied by the CO). This will help you determine the standard you need to achieve in this subject.

The CO provide information under three headings: fitness to practise, nature of the examination and assessment.

Fitness to practise

To be able to carry out the full range of contact lens work requires further training and a depth of experience, which cannot be expected of a newly registered optometrist.

On first registration, however, optometrists must be competent to safely advise prospective wearers of their suitability for contact lenses, to prescribe and fit basic forms of contact lenses, to provide aftercare in such cases, and to provide competent advice to habitual wearers. Above all, however, they must recognize their limitations in this field of optometry and be ready to refer patients whose contact lens problems are beyond their competence to colleagues qualified to provide a specialized service.

Candidates must demonstrate an adequate standard of knowledge and skill to enable them to deal safely with contact lens cases with regard to:

- Observation of the patient
- Handling contact lenses
- The relevant basic science

- Managing and advising patients
- Candidates' basic knowledge must be seen as more important than the extent of their experience.

Nature of the examination

The examination lasts for 90 minutes and is with two examiners. It is in two parts.

(i) Practical fitting session

This part will last for 45 minutes. The candidate is provided with a patient and should be advised that the patient is a prospective contact lens wearer, and that it may be assumed that a full preliminary routine, including a slit lamp and keratometry, has been carried out. The candidate should then be required to:

(a) Carry out whatever further measurements are considered necessary to a contact lens case
(b) Select a suitable rigid and soft lens type on the basis of the available information
(c) Insert a rigid and soft lens
(d) Make an assessment of lens fit and performance, suggest suitable modifications to improve fit and be prepared to discuss the suggestions
(e) Specify an order for the required contact lenses
(f) Demonstrate knowledge of contact lens dispensing, instructions and advice to accompany initial lens supply.

(ii) Practical aftercare and oral section

This part of the examination will also last 45 minutes and is with a different examiner. This section should emphasize the importance of continuing clinical care. The candidate should be prepared to examine a patient who is a contact lens wearer; slides may also be available. The candidate should be required to:

(a) Take the symptoms and history of the patient
(b) Carry out a suitable examination of the patient to determine the effects of contact lens wear on the ocular integrity; ideally contact lens related phenomena should be observed by use of a slit lamp
(c) Determine the lens care regimen and patient compliance with lens hygiene and storage recommendations
(d) Discuss the need for remedial action and advise the patient accordingly.

The candidate should be required to demonstrate through discussion:

(a) An understanding of the principles and importance of taking a patient's symptoms and history

(b) An understanding of lens modification, and the properties of lens materials and care solutions, for this may be applied to problem solving or alleviation of adverse reactions to lens wear
(c) The ability to give appropriate advice to habitual and prospective lens wearers who may be the primary responsibility of the practitioner
(d) A knowledge of the legal regulations relevant to contact lens practice.

In all parts of the examination the examiner may go beyond the points listed, should it be thought necessary to do so to establish the candidate's fitness to practise within the limitations of the syllabus.

Assessment

In every case the examiners will look to see that candidates have adequate ability in basic fitting and aftercare techniques in order to manage contact lens patients safely.
Candidates should:

(i) Complete procedures in an orderly manner
(ii) Demonstrate a command of basic knowledge and techniques in order to make valid decisions
(iii) Make correct appraisals of significant signs and symptoms
(iv) Recognize their own present limitations in contact lens practice.

16.2 THE EXAMINATION FORMAT

The fitting and aftercare/oral sections may occur in either order. For the aftercare section you are likely to be told to go through your normal routine but to talk through and describe what you are observing and why you are doing various tests. It is likely that the examiner will stop and question you at various stages throughout your routine and also tell you to skip various procedures, e.g. ophthalmoscopy, after you have stated that you are about to do it. Make sure you have practised a set routine so that you know exactly which step you are going to do next. Important procedures are less likely to be missed out with good preparation.

For the fitting session you will be asked to insert a rigid and a soft lens. Make sure that you can justify which should be inserted first. Be aware that the 'K' readings given by the examiners may not actually be accurate, therefore if the fit of your lens looks abnormally steep or flat, don't be afraid to say so! Also, the lens packet could be marked with the wrong specifications! It is important to know in detail your lenses of choice, particularly the parameters available, so you can suggest alternative specifications should the fit not be ideal. The type of slit lamp and the fitting sets found at each examination centre will vary – find out what will be available from other pre-registration optometrists who have studied at the department, or from the centre itself if you are sitting the exam in unfamiliar territory. You may take your own fitting sets with you if you prefer, but if you do then make sure you know everything you can about the lenses. Also be familiar with a few alternatives, just in case you are presented with a patient whose characteristics do not match the parameters you have brought with you, e.g. if they have a very small or large corneal diameter.

16.3 WHAT DO THE EXAMINERS SAY?

(a) Advice to candidates preparing for the exam

Gain as much experience in as broad a selection of lens types as possible during your pre-registration year. If your practice does not have many contact lens patients then make arrangements to visit another practice and/or hospital department to gain more practical knowledge. Read the contact lens articles in *OT* and the *Optician* and textbooks to keep up with new developments of lenses and solutions. A good source of information about current lenses is *The International Contact Lens Yearbook*.

Ensure that you are very familiar with the types of lenses and solutions you use in practice and be able to state the reasons why you use each particular product. Try to sit in with an experienced practitioner and observe fitting and management and also get them to sit in with you to comment on how your technique can be improved. Adopt a good aftercare/fitting routine from an early stage and familiarize yourself with handling lenses and inserting and removing them from the eye.

(b) Areas of the subject that require sound knowledge

These include:

(i)   The ability to recognize ocular changes caused by contact lenses, and the urgency with which remedial action should be taken and when to refer on

(ii) Being able to demonstrate how to handle contact lenses and insert and remove them from the eye

(iii) Basic contact lens fitting and what constitutes a 'good' or 'bad' fit

(iv) Hygiene

(v)   A very good slit lamp routine.

(c) What is looked for in a successful candidate?

The examiners are looking for a safe common-sense approach with the ability to think logically and make good decisions. The candidate should show an understanding of the links between various signs, symptoms and procedures, and be able to explain findings and state what actions should be taken and why.

The candidate should appear well-organized and possess good clinical and inter-personal communication skills with the ability to handle lenses competently. They must also have sound background knowledge.

(d) and (e) Things which bring marks down and common causes of failure
This can include general lack of knowledge of lens types/solutions available, poor management and understanding of dangerous signs or symptoms, disorganized and disjointed routines, poor slit lamp technique, lack of awareness of one's own limitations, poor observation, obvious lack of contact lens experience, poor hygiene, and generally appearing unsafe.

(f) Subject areas that candidates place too little importance on
Areas examiners often feel candidates should place more importance on include the law relating to contact lens practice and optometric responsibilities, practical ability, lens recognition and verification, the ability to manage complications, contact lens solutions, and the optics of contact lenses.

16.4 HELP AND ADVICE

During the pre-registration year try to get as much experience as possible. Talk to other optometrists, contact lens opticians and pre-registration optometrists about the lenses they use. Be aware of the range of lenses and solutions available that may not be found in practice. If you find your practice does not have a great number of contact lens patients, take action as early in the pre-registration year as possible to get the extra experience required, e.g. observe in contact lens clinics on a regular basis or arrange a 'practice-swap' with another pre-registration optometrist.

Contact lens practice is considered by some authorities to be more of an art than a science, and great importance is placed on practical ability and patient handling skills. So make sure you have the opportunity to acquire them.

During the exam you may be asked about your 'first-choice' lenses in great detail. Find out as much as you can, e.g. method of manufacture, material constituents, Dk, optic zone diameters and peripheral curves, available parameters, and solution contra-indications. Telephone the contact lens and solution manufacturers and ask them to send full details of their products (rather than just advertising leaflets).

Try also to become familiar with as much equipment as possible, especially slit lamps. During the examination there is usually a choice of Haag Streit or Zeiss types but be prepared to use either if necessary. Develop a good slit lamp technique, i.e. set the eyepieces, adjust the height of the table to make the patient comfortable, adjust the chin rest to line up the eye with the canthus markers, try to minimize the discomfort caused by glare and observe the eyes and contact lenses in a logical manner. Practise lid eversion on as many contact lens patients as possible. For the various slit lamps, also be aware of the amount of magnification produced and its limitations, what the various filters can be used for, and the best method of illumination to observe various features of the eye and contact lens.

It is important to develop a proper routine for aftercare and fitting from an early stage. It is obvious to examiners which candidates have not been used to contact lens patients. During the exam, your people-handling skills will be closely observed. Although you may be nervous, do make an effort to put the patient at ease and don't treat them like a piece of equipment. Good hygiene is essential; ensure you wash your hands and clean/lubricate any trial lenses before insertion if this has not already been done.

Be aware that a couple of common tasks may be set during the examination. Examples include: to measure the BOZR of a rigid lens with a radiuscope, or to write down full specifications of a rigid lens in a 'tricurve' design after the skeleton parameters have been given.

Slides may be shown of various contact lens related disorders. Make sure you can recognize common lens wear complications and know the management of them in practice. This includes knowing when to refer or inform the GP.

Useful equipment to take: trial frame, ruler with gauge to measure horizontal visible iris diameter, interpalpebral aperture and pupil sizes, cotton buds (or equivalent) for lid eversion, V gauge and contact lens focimeter attachment.

16.5 PAST EXAM QUESTIONS

1 How does the pH of saline differ from that of tears?
2 What is the difference between follicles and papillae?
3 What advice/action is necessary for a contact lens wearer who had contact lens associated papillary conjunctivitis?
4 How would you grade the different stages of papillae presence in contact lens associated papillary conjunctivitis?
5 Would you use fluorescein during contact lens aftercare?
6 Is it necessary to perform ophthalmoscopy during routine contact lens aftercare?
7 What lenses have you used in practice?
8 What methods are used to manufacture contact lenses?
9 What are the advantages and disadvantages of each method of manufacture?
10 What substances are added to rigid lenses to improve: (i) oxygen transmission, (ii) wettability. Are there any undesirable characteristics produced by these substances?
11 How does altering the radius of a rigid/soft lens affect the power?
12 Does altering the diameter of a rigid/soft lens necessitate changing other parameters to give an equivalent fit?
13 What modifications can be made to contact lenses?
14 Can the lenses chosen during a previous fitting session be modified in any way?

15 What percentage of protein does a protein tablet remove?

16 What are the main categories of cleaning/disinfecting solutions?

17 What care system would you recommend as first choice for: (i) soft lenses, (ii) hard lenses, (iii) rigid gas permeable lenses (RGP)? Why would you choose these particular types?

18 What advice would you give to a contact lens wearer who is taking medication in the form of eye drops?

19 What type of contact lenses (if any) would you recommend for an atopic patient?

20 Should diabetics be fitted with contact lenses?

21 What product is used by manufacturers to polish rigid lenses?

22 Would you fit a patient with contact lenses on an 'extended wear' basis? If so, what follow-up management would you use?

23 What does 'Dk' mean?

24 What is the Dk of various different lenses?

25 What are 'SEALS'? How should they be managed?

26 What causes 3 and 9 o'clock staining? How can it be alleviated?

27 What are with the rule and against the rule astigmatism?

28 Is iris colour related to corneal sensitivity?

29 What is the maximum wearing time you would recommend for contact lenses?

30 What follow-up criteria do you recommend for a new lens wearer?

31 What contra-indications are there to contact lens wear?

32 What methods can be used to assess the tear film in practice?

33 What is a 'normal' tear break up time?

34 If a patient appeared to have a low tear volume, what type of contact lens material would you choose?

35 Is the Schirmer test a good predictor of tear volume?

36 What advice would you give regarding the disinfections of contact lens cases?

37 If an RGP wearer required new spectacles how long would you advise that lenses are kept out before a spectacle refraction is performed? Are there any complications?

38 If a patient brought in a contact lens prescription from another practice, would you order a duplicate lens? What is the legal criterion used?

39 What does 'buffered' mean in terms of saline?

40 Are all-in-one solutions better than their predecessors?

41 What type of contact lenses can be used to correct presbyopia?

42 What methods of construction are used to stabilize soft toric contact lenses?

43 What are jelly bumps? Can they be removed from a lens? How is the formation of jelly bumps best prevented?

44 Are rust spots on contact lenses a problem?

45 Is it safe to go swimming while wearing contact lenses?

46 What is the minimum magnification necessary to observe the corneal endothelium?

47 What action would you take if you observed early corneal vascularization with a habitual soft lens wearer?

48 What advice would you give regarding lens disinfection to a patient who wears their lenses on a very occasional basis?

49 What advice would you give regarding the wearing time for an occasional lens wearer?

50 What is the difference between sterilizing and disinfecting a contact lens?

51 How would you manage a person with marginal keratitis?

52 How would you manage a patient with a corneal ulcer?

53 What contact lens options are available to the presbyope?

54 What criteria would you use for selecting a patient for monovision?

55 What parameters are available in daily disposable contact lenses?

56 What are the clinical signs of Meibomian gland dysfunction?

57 What clinical tests would you use to assess symptoms of dry eyes?

58 What treatments are available for dry eyes?

59 What materials are extended wear contact lenses made from and which types of patient are suitable for fitting?

60 How does pregnancy affect contact lens wear?

16.6 MORE INFO?

Efron, N. *Contact Lens Complications*, second edition. Oxford: Butterworth-Heinemann, 2004.

Efron, N. *Contact Lens Practice*. Oxford: Butterworth-Heinemann, 2002

Jones, L and Jones, D. *Common Contact Lens Complications: Diagnosis and Management*. Oxford: Butterworth-Heinemann, 2000.

Gasson, A and Morris, J. *The Contact Lens Manual: A Practical Guide to Fitting*, third edition. Oxford: Butterworth-Heinemann, 2003.

Veys, J, Meyler, J and Davies, I. *Essential Contact Lens Practice: A Practical Guide*. Oxford: Butterworth-Heinemann, 2002.

Phillips, AJ and Speedwell, P. *Contact Lenses*, fourth edition. Oxford: Butterworth-Heinemann, 1997.

Useful addresses

Division of Optometry
Aston University
Aston Triangle
Birmingham B4 7ET
0121 359 3611
www.aston.ac.uk

Department of Optometry
University of Bradford
Richmond Road
Bradford
West Yorkshire BD7 1DP
01274 234640
http://www.brad.ac.uk/university/ugpros/optometry.php
optometry-enquiries@bradford.ac.uk

The Department of Optometry and Visual Science
City University
Northampton Square
London EC1V 0HB
020 7040 8339
http://www.city.ac.uk/optometry/
Clinical facilities are at
The Department of Optometry and Visual Science
7–9 Bath Street
London EC1V 9LF

Department of Vision Sciences
Glasgow Caledonian University
City Campus
Cowcaddens Road
Glasgow G4 0BA
Scotland
0141 331 3000
Vision.Sciences@gcal.ac.uk
http://www.vis.gcal.ac.uk/

Department of Optometry and Vision Sciences
Cardiff University
Redwood Building
King Edward VII Avenue
Cathays Park
Cardiff CF10 3NB
029 2087 4852
http://www.cf.ac.uk/optom/

Optometry and Neuroscience
UMIST
Sackville Street
Manchester, UK
M60 1QD
0161 200 3870
joanne.cohen@umist.ac.uk
http://www2.umist.ac.uk/optometry/

School of Biomedical Sciences
University of Ulster at Coleraine
Cromore Road
Co Londonderry
BT52 1SA
08 700 400 700
online@ulster.ac.uk
http://www.ulst.ac.uk/

Department of Optometry and Ophthalmic Dispensing
School of Applied Sciences
Anglia Polytechnic University
East Road
Cambridge CB1 1PT
01223 363271
http://www.apu.ac.uk/appsci/optometry/index.html

Association of Optometrists
61 Southwark Street
London SE1 0HL
020 7261 9661
postbox@assoc-optometrists.org
http://www.assoc-optometrists.org
http://www.assoc-optometrists.org/student/prereg_learning_scheme.html for a series of
typical PQE questions and answers

The College of Optometrists
42 Craven Street
London WC2N 5NG
020 7839 6000
pre_reg@College-optometrists.org

General Optical Council
41 Harley Street
London W1N 2DJ
020 7580 3898
goc@optical.org
http:/www.optical.org

Institute of Optometry
56–62, Newington Causeway
London SE1 6DS
020 7407 4183
admin@ioo.org.uk
http://www.ioo.org.uk/

The Orthoptic and Binocular Vision Association
4 Church Street
Tamworth
Staffordshire B79 7DE
Tel: 01827 61600
(The OBVA organize annual courses for the Binocular Vision PQE that are held in early
March at Aston University)

Hirji Associates
Consulting in Optometry
7 Milford Road
Harborne
Birmingham B17 9RL
0121 682 7041
info@hirji.co.uk
http://www.hirji.co.uk/

For information on CHESAS
JCL Consulting
PO Box 336
Beckenham
BR3 4UZ
http://www.jclconsulting.co.uk

Index

appeal procedures 29
application forms, completing 8–9
assessment 50, 61, 68, 82, 95, 106, 117, 126,
    137

CV 4
  writing 6ff
case records 120
communication skills 39ff
courses 35–6
cover letter 4

equipment 19, 129
examination
  advice for practical 97
  counselling after failure 29
  equipment for practical 54, 129
  format 51, 62, 69, 75, 82, 107, 118, 126,
    137
  oral 55, 94, 101, 130
  overseas candidates 29–30
  technique 37
examiners, training of 26

HES 9ff
hospital practice 33

illumination 87

independent practice 12ff
interviews 17ff

law 121
lighting 87
lighting levels 88

model routine 111
multiple practice 15ff

non-verbal behaviour 40–2

pre-registration year 22–5, 32–3
protection 89

responsibilities 90
re-takes 27–8, 45–6
rumours about PQEs 28–30

slit lamp 70, 72
study groups 34

tonometry 70, 71–2

VTA 85
venues 37
verbal behaviour 42–4
vision screening 86–7